10 Simple Solutions to Chronic Pa *a fulfilling life while living with pa change pain sufferers into people abl easy-to-understand language, with cu...* *examples, this book provides readers with tools to more effectively manage their pain. The suggestions and strategies in this book are well-reasoned, practical, and easily accomplished by those wanting mastery over pain.*

> —B. Eliot Cole, MD, MPA, executive director of the American Society of Pain Educators

Victims of chronic pain will find help in this research-based yet easily understood book. Tearnan engages the reader as an active member of the pain-treatment team. This proven program works to effectively reduce pain and suffering.

> —C. David Tollison, Ph.D., author and editor of eleven textbooks on the diagnosis and interdisciplinary treatment of pain and recipient of numerous national awards for the research and treatment of pain

Tearnan's book is a well written, practical patient guide to chronic pain management. Reading this informative book will give chronic pain patients greater insight and helpful techniques to more effectively manage their pain.

> —Steven Berman, MD, medical director of the Functional Restoration Program Renown Rehabilitation Hospital, Reno, NV

10 Simple Solutions to Chronic Pain

How to Stop Pain from Controlling Your Life

BLAKE H. TEARNAN, PH.D.

New Harbinger Publications, Inc.

Publisher's Note

This publication is designed to provide accurate and authoritative information in regard to the subject matter covered. It is sold with the understanding that the publisher is not engaged in rendering psychological, financial, legal, or other professional services. If expert assistance or counseling is needed, the services of a competent professional should be sought.

Care has been taken to confirm the accuracy of the information presented and to describe generally accepted practices. However, the authors, editors, and publisher are not responsible for errors or omissions or for any consequences from application of the information in this book and make no warranty, express or implied, with respect to the contents of the publication.

The authors, editors, and publisher have exerted every effort to ensure that any drug selection and dosage set forth in this text are in accordance with current recommendations and practice at the time of publication. However, in view of ongoing research, changes in government regulations, and the constant flow of information relating to drug therapy and drug reactions, the reader is urged to check the package insert for each drug for any change in indications and dosage and for added warnings and precautions. This is particularly important when the recommended agent is a new or infrequently employed drug.

Some drugs and medical devices presented in this publication may have Food and Drug Administration (FDA) clearance for limited use in restricted research settings. It is the responsibility of the health care provider to ascertain the FDA status of each drug or device planned for use in their clinical practice.

Acquired by Jess O'Brien; Cover design by Amy Shoup;
Edited by Jasmine Star; Text design by Tracy Carlson

Library of Congress Cataloging-in-Publication Data

Tearnan, Blake H.

10 simple solutions to chronic pain : how to stop pain from controlling your life / Blake H. Tearnan.

p. cm.

Includes bibliographical references and index.

ISBN-13: 978-1-57224-482-5 (alk. paper)

ISBN-10: 1-57224-482-8 (alk. paper) 40522319 6/09

1. Chronic pain--Popular works. 2. Chronic pain--Treatment--Popular works. 3. Chronic pain--Psychological aspects--Popular works. I. Title. II. Title: Ten simple solutions to chronic pain.

RB127.T39 2007

616'.0472--dc22

2007005760

09 08 07   10 9 8 7 6 5 4 3 2 1   First printing

This book is dedicated to all of my patients, who have taught me the most about the enormous capacity of the human spirit to live successfully with pain.

Contents

Foreword

With the great prevalence of chronic pain in this country and associated health care costs estimated to be $80 billion each year, there is a growing need for effective chronic pain management. Fortunately, a newer approach has proven to be effective, both therapeutically and in terms of cost. Based on the biopsychosocial model of pain, this orientation emphasizes the importance of taking into account the dynamic interplay among biological, psychological, and social factors in better understanding and treating chronic pain.

Unlike earlier approaches, which mostly aimed to ease symptoms, the biopsychosocial approach emphasizes the active role patients are expected to play in the treatment process. In a sense, the health care provider serves as a coach who helps engender self-management and coping skills in patients with chronic pain. The patient and the health care provider actively work together to meet the important goals of increasing functioning, managing pain, and setting reasonable goals in order to return to an appropriate level of day-to-day activities.

People suffering from chronic pain need to be fully educated about the process of managing their pain, including the often complex factors that interact to maintain and even exacerbate chronic pain. Dr. Tearnan's book is a condensed library of knowledge covering the basic important information you need to understand about pain, and providing concrete and easy-to-implement techniques to make you an active participant in your pain-management process.

Dr. Tearnan will help you understand the emotional component of pain and how it relates to anxiety and a sense of threat, as well as the role of negative thoughts in maintaining chronic pain. He details methods of changing pain behaviors, enhancing your general well-being, and dealing with family issues that can arise from chronic pain. You'll also learn effective methods for increasing your activity level and monitoring your progress. Dr. Tearnan provides basic information about sleep, medications, and traditional medical procedures (such as physical therapies, massage, chiropractic manipulation, injection therapies, and surgical treatments), which will allow you to intelligently interact with health care professionals when attempting to glean more reliable and valid information about your condition. Case histories provide additional perspective and illustrate how others have benefited from the techniques outlined in the book. And exercises provided throughout the book will help you put the techniques to work to help with your own chronic pain. Again, this is important because it reinforces the key role you must play in your pain management program.

Knowledge is power. With the great wealth of information and techniques presented in this book, you'll increase your power and be better able to manage your chronic pain.

—Robert J. Gatchel, Ph.D., ABPP
Department Chairman, Department of Psychology
University of Texas at Arlington

Acknowledgments

I would like to thank the many people who supported me in writing this book. First, and foremost, thanks to my wife, Olivia, for reading the various drafts of the manuscript and giving me invaluable feedback. This thanks also extends to my daughters, Audrey and Vanessa, for reading some of the chapters and putting up with me in my long hours of isolation. I would also like to thank Donna Alexander of St. Mary's Hospital in Reno for her invaluable assistance in gathering important research papers for my review. Thanks also to my transcriptionist, Janis Lamers, for deciphering my garbled dictation. My gratitude also to Jess O'Brien at New Harbinger Publications for his patience and to the various editors at New Harbinger Publications for their careful attention to detail and guidance in the writing. I am also grateful to my colleagues at Washoe Medical Center for their professional collaboration, including Steve Berman, MD, Ken Pitman, MD, Andrew Wesley, MD, Steve Igaz, MA, Cathy Kline, MA, and P. J. Juhrend, MA. Finally, a special thanks to Dr. William Tao for his friendship and support.

Introduction

Chronic pain affects 50 million Americans (Gatchel and Turk 1996), with nearly 11.7 million individuals disabled by back pain alone (Holbrook et al. 1984). The impacts of chronic pain can be devastating—loss of job and income, disruption of family life, general physical decline, disturbance of sleep, depression, social isolation, and dependence on narcotics.

Chronic pain is now recognized as a serious problem by most physicians and medical schools, and residency programs are devoting more time to teaching doctors to diagnose and treat chronic pain. New technologies to help with pain continue to emerge, including medications and surgical techniques that would have been unthinkable fifty years ago. However, despite these advances, more people than ever are disabled by pain, and the cost, especially in terms of human suffering, continues to escalate.

Nearly twenty years ago, Dr. Wilber Fordyce, a well-known pain psychologist and researcher at the University of Washington, wrote that the most important question patients can ask when they're first injured is "Why am I in pain?" (1988). This orients patients and doctors toward investigating the underlying cause of the pain and dedicating their efforts to curing the problem.

But Dr. Fordyce also asserted that if pain has been unremitting for three months or longer, the most important question patients can start to ask is "Why am I suffering?" Certainly, part of the reason is physical, whether due to a damaged nerve, scar tissue, disc pain, or a host of other reasons.

However, a large part of the reason why people with persistent pain suffer and are disabled is because they're fearful, caught in a losing cycle of boom-and-bust attempts to increase activity, crippled by uncertainties about their future, fatigued by ineffective and risky treatments, and confused by a medical system that often fails to provide needed direction to patients. Feeling helpless, individuals sometimes turn to desperate means to alleviate their discomfort.

Trying to cure the problem of chronic pain is sometimes not the solution but the problem. Instead, pain experts in recent years have recommended that teaching people to live with pain, to improve their quality of life despite pain, is the best approach to help individuals live fuller and happier lives. This new approach is not a pull-yourself-up-by-your-bootstraps cry to action, too often the only message people hear when told by their doctors, "You're going to have to live with your pain." Rather, it's a hopeful approach that encourages individuals to get off the roller-coaster ride of medical treatments that simply do not work and instead leave most people feeling more discouraged.

I am affiliated with two pain programs, one in Reno (Washoe Medical Center Rehabilitation Hospital) and the other in Las Vegas, Nevada (Southern Nevada Functional Restoration Program). Both are staffed by psychologists, physicians, and physical and occupational therapists. The goal of both programs is to teach patients better coping skills for managing their pain and improving the quality of their lives. We see patients on an individual basis, but most participate in a four-week program consisting of daily physical and occupational therapy, sessions with the psychologist to improve coping skills, wellness classes to address various aspects of living with pain, and weekly physician visits.

As with other comprehensive approaches to managing pain, our programs rarely eliminate pain altogether. But almost without exception, if patients put forth even minimal effort they leave feeling more confident and hopeful about the future, and with a renewed desire to live life again to its fullest. I've also developed a Web site, HealthNetSolutions.com, where you can learn more about pain assessment and assess your own pain and disability. Although the Web site is designed primarily for pain professionals, all are welcome.

Who Should Read This Book

If you've struggled with pain and find yourself with little hope and exhausted from the daily misery of wondering what's around the corner, this book is written for you. It offers a renewed sense of promise and direction, not by means of simple platitudes that things will get better, but rather by taking you on a journey of discovery. You'll learn how to manage and deal more effectively with life even if you can't eliminate your pain. The goal is to put you back in control of your life and help you become more certain about your future and ready for the challenges you face with pain. This will require hard work and patience, qualities you most likely believe you lack after so many months and even years of suffering with pain and experiencing so many failures. However, the journey starts with small steps and the obstacles to getting better are not insurmountable, no matter how long you've suffered.

Many of my patients believe that letting go of the hope for a cure for their pain, no matter how elusive, is admitting to failure, resigning to the ravages of pain without hope and happiness. Not so. You can live with pain and learn to be happy, but you need to be willing to take a different path—one that has been traveled by thousands of people with chronic pain who are living normal and successful lives. If you're ready to try something different, to see the problem of pain in a new light, this book will help you.

How This Book Can Help

Can a self-help book on chronic pain really change your life for the better? There are a lot of books about pain, and most offer good advice about different medical treatments available to patients. This information is useful, especially when people are confronted with a dizzying array of concoctions, techniques, procedures, and new surgical advances. This book is different. It focuses more on how to cope and adapt so you can live a full life despite pain. The strategies described, which incorporate the latest knowledge on the treatment of chronic pain, are well researched and used by major pain clinics across the country. These treatments are usually carried out by a team of clinicians consisting of a psychologist, a physician, a physical therapist, and sometimes an occupational therapist. However, self-help books that provide useful information and teach better skills for dealing with pain have also proven effective.

This book will not cure or eliminate your pain, but it will help you cope with pain better. And if you follow its strategies, you will reduce your suffering and disability. With a little work, the application of knowledge-based skills, and the right choices, you can improve your activity level, sleep, mood, and overall quality of life. You just need to practice the strategies described. Reading this book will also help you interact more effectively with your doctors and other health care providers by giving you the knowledge to take charge of your health. It will help you ask better questions, be comfortable saying no to treatments that might be harmful or ineffective, and request care you believe you need. Studies have shown that when people are more informed and involved in the management of their pain, they feel better and are more satisfied (Gatchel 2005).

This simple and straightforward book offers practical advice for managing chronic pain better. There are other texts that are much longer and go into greater detail, especially about the physical mechanisms believed to underlie many pain problems. Some of these are listed in the section Recommended Readings at the end of the book.

Learning is not like a light switch. You should expect some ups and downs on your journey, and sometimes you will get discouraged. However, if your goals are clear and you're willing to go back to the drawing board, sometimes several times, you will experience significant changes that will prove long lasting.

It will be useful for you to keep a journal as you read this book. This will help you monitor your progress and provide a place for you to write down things you need to remember. Taking notes and recording your experiences reinforces what you learn and helps you share what you've learned with loved ones and your doctors.

You'll also need a journal to complete the exercises in this book. It's important to do each exercise, since they're designed to strengthen the knowledge and skills you'll gain as you read through this book. Write your responses in your journal so you can refer to your answers later.

With hard work and a willingness to try—especially when things seem the toughest—you should see significant changes in just a few weeks. Remember, it isn't just the special few who succeed in managing pain better; everyone is capable of positive changes. But success depends on practice, realistic expectations, and a willingness to get back on the horse. If you set yourself to the task, you will achieve your goals of feeling significantly better and gaining control of your life once again.

Tips for Success

The outcome of treatments for chronic pain depends on the amount of effort you put forth. If you don't do anything, it's unlikely that your situation will improve. But most people will benefit if they commit to even minimal effort. In our treatment program in Reno, about 85 percent of patients improve, 60 percent significantly. Here are some of the reasons people succeed:

- Willingness to put aside anger and mistrust

- Deemphasizing pain relief above all else as a measure of success

- Active instead of passive involvement in the program

- Willingness to explore the behavioral and psychological management of pain

- Compliance with therapeutic recommendations, especially in relation to increasing activity level

- Taking ownership of their therapeutic program

- Willingness to move toward a reduction and possibly elimination of narcotic analgesics

- Taking steps to reduce fears of pain and its consequences by engaging in physical activity and confronting nonproductive beliefs

- Willingness to accept pain as an ongoing experience and letting go of a cure

Learning to live with pain means learning to live your life differently. It means developing skills and knowledge, not to fight pain better, but to meet the challenges of pain without fear and uncertainty—the true enemies that can lead to the increased suffering and disabling consequences that affect so many millions of people with chronic pain. This book will help you find a new perspective on your pain problem and offer you specific techniques for learning to live with and manage your chronic pain.

1

Understanding Pain and Suffering

Learning more about pain, and specifically about the interrelationship between pain, suffering, and disability, will allow you to better understand your own situation. This is an important first step in learning how to manage your pain and improve your quality of life. It's also the foundation for understanding and implementing all of the solutions in the chapters that follow.

Pain arises from actual or potential damage to the body, motivating people to take action to avoid harm or seek recuperation (Asmundson 1999). Cognitive and emotional factors come into play as the pain information enters the central nervous system. How a person interprets and responds to pain is influenced by the expected threat associated with the pain.

Defining Pain

Pain is difficult to define since it's something we can't touch or see. It's a subjective experience, and it's also basic to our survival. As you'll learn, pain is much more than the feeling you get when you stub your toe or burn yourself on a hot stove.

How we define pain is important, since it helps to make this complex experience more understandable, leading to better ways of approaching solutions to the problem of pain. In 1982, pain expert John Loeser proposed that pain consists of four dimensions: nociception, pain, suffering, and pain behavior. "Nociception" is a complicated-sounding word, but it simply refers to potential tissue damage and injury that excites nerve endings. Think of *nociception* as the underlying physical mechanism that initiates the signal of pain. The second dimension, *pain*, is the sensation experienced as a consequence of nociception. Subjectively, you might describe your pain as achy, tender, sore, sharp, stabbing, or burning. *Suffering* is the negative emotion generated by pain and problems associated with pain, such as stress and various losses. Finally, *pain behavior* refers to any behavior you exhibit in association with the presence of pain, such as facial expressions, speech patterns, taking medication, asking others for help, and limiting your activities.

Loeser's view of pain is a useful starting point. However, the components need to be understood in a broader context, especially with regard to how you interpret and react to pain, and how your pain is affected by various social influences and other environmental factors. In other words, pain is not simply a well-defined response to a physical stimulus registered in the central nervous system and resulting in an uncomfortable sensation. As nociceptive stimulation enters the spinal cord and brain, the signal doesn't travel to a specific pain center. Pain information travels to many areas of the brain involved with interpretation, judgment, and emotions. This is where matters get complex, since distraction, past experiences with pain, fears attributed to pain, perception of coping strength, social support, and a whole host of other factors determine in a puzzling way how pain is experienced and how you respond to it.

Historically, pain has been thought of in purely mechanistic terms. The analogy often used for pain is a rope and a bell—a jerk of the rope causes the pain bell to ring. However, this is too simplistic. For example, it doesn't account for why people who are anxious experience more intense pain. The experience of pain is affected by a variety of psychological, social, and cultural influences, calling into question the notion that pain can be adequately explained by a wired, mechanistic process.

Acute Versus Chronic Pain

Acute pain refers to pain that lasts less than three months. Acute pain serves a useful purpose, helping motivate us to take action to protect ourselves. Tissue damage, swelling, and inflammation are characteristic of new-onset pain. Normally, but not always, the extent of the damage determines the intensity of pain experienced. Acute pain is generally responsive to treatment, such as medications. Emotionally, acute pain can trigger feelings of anxiety, which is usually a good thing because anxiety helps motivate us to take action, such as seeking help, monitoring the status of the injury, and being careful to avoid further injury.

In the 1970s, most pain experts used six months as the dividing point between acute and chronic pain. However, research now shows that it takes much less time for the majority of injuries to heal. Your body is very adept at marshaling its defenses and doing what's necessary to promote healing, and after three months most healing is complete. Injured disks, recovery from certain surgeries, and other exceptional problems may take longer to heal.

Chronic pain is a condition where pain has been persistent for three months or longer, well past the time for normal healing. No longer useful, the pain simply interferes with day-to-day activities and life in general (Turk and Winter 2006). Chronic pain is usually constant, but it can also be episodic or recurrent, as in headaches. Pain intensity can vary considerably and, as you'll learn, it can be affected by a variety of physical, environmental, social, and psychological factors.

Models of Pain

Models are ways of organizing and understanding complex phenomena, and doctors and others use models to explain the puzzle of pain. Models also have a tremendous influence on how doctors try to solve the problem of pain.

DISEASE MODEL

The *disease model* assumes a person's pain complaints can be explained, in essence, by some specific disease state. Treatment interventions are aimed at correcting the physical cause of pain. The model is simple, which makes it attractive. However, despite advances in anatomy and all of the medical sciences, there's general agreement that physical factors alone cannot adequately explain the problem of pain (Turk and Monarch 2002).

GATE CONTROL THEORY

In 1965, Melzack and Wall proposed the *gate control theory* of pain. They hypothesized that there's a gating mechanism in the spinal cord that moderates pain, and that the gate can open or close due to a number of physical as well as psychological factors. Anxiety, negative thinking, and focusing on the pain, for example, can open the gate. Relaxation, positive emotions, and distraction, on the other hand, can close it.

At the time it was proposed, the gate control theory was revolutionary since it argued that pain is not a one-way street that acts like a rope and bell. Pain is modulated as it enters the spinal cord and is altered significantly more as it's registered in the brain. It's affected by a variety of factors, such as how you interpret the pain and relate it to past experiences. Pain perception is also affected by any threat attached to pain. In this model, if you've coped successfully with pain in the past and the symptoms you're experiencing can be explained in relatively benign terms, you're less likely to react as strongly, both emotionally and physically. The disease model doesn't take these complex factors into account.

Although there's uncertainty as to the exact nature of the "gate" and its location in the central nervous system, the theory was particularly important when it was proposed, since it allows for a variety of factors to influence pain, especially psychological events. It helped to alter the way pain experts thought about pain, especially by drawing attention to the shortcomings of the disease model, and it paved the way for the now generally accepted view of pain, the biopsychosocial model of pain.

BIOPSYCHOSOCIAL MODEL OF PAIN

As researchers became increasingly convinced that the experience of pain, especially chronic pain, was a complex synergy of physical, social, behavioral, emotional, and environmental influences, a new model emerged—the *biopsychosocial model*. George Engel (1977) first proposed this term to argue that all medical problems, not just those associated with pain, are influenced by biological, psychological, and social factors. Diabetes, for example, has an obvious biological basis involving the pancreas. However, the ways in which people relate to a diagnosis of diabetes—the steps they take in managing the disease and how they respond to various social influences—determine in an interactive fashion the course and outcome of their illness. Isolating one factor and using it to explain diabetes, according to Engel, doesn't capture the complex nature of the disease. Medical problems are multidimensional and affected by many factors, and so is pain.

Current research has clearly shown that the most effective methods for managing the problems of chronic pain take into account the multiple factors influencing pain, giving due respect to the biological basis of pain but not ignoring other aspects that are often more influential, such as psychological and social factors. The biopsychosocial model is the approach used to guide this book.

Exercise: Understanding Your Chronic Pain

Now that you've learned some background information about pain and suffering, take some time to answer the following questions. Write your responses in your journal so you can refer to them later:

1. The biopsychosocial model emphasizes the multidimensional nature of pain. Biological factors alone cannot account for the experience of pain. Do you believe your pain is influenced by social and psychological events? How does your pain change when you feel angry or stressed?

2. The amount of damage to your body and the pain you feel aren't directly proportional. In other words, hurt and harm

are not the same in chronic pain. What does this mean in terms of your pain?

3. Suffering is the misery associated with your pain. What are the reasons you're suffering other than your pain? Do you think it's possible to change these things without eliminating your pain?

Physical and Nonphysical Factors in Chronic Pain

Although the healing of the original injury is usually complete in chronic, nonmalignant pain, that doesn't mean that there's no underlying physical condition causing pain. Multiple mechanisms that may produce pain are often present after healing, such as nerve irritation, tense muscles and ligaments, and changes in joints. Unfortunately, modern medicine has no definitive way of sorting out how much any one of these potential causes might be contributing to the experience of pain.

For example, consider low back pain. The most common pain problem, it afflicts over two-thirds of people with chronic disabling pain, yet it's still poorly understood. Nearly 85 percent of those with back pain receive a *nonspecific diagnosis*, meaning that no definitive physical cause of the pain is known (Gatchel 2005). Back pain could arise from a number of sources, including muscles, ligaments, joints, disks, or nerve roots. The cause is usually only clear if the person has a fracture, tumor, or infection. In only 15 percent of cases can physicians pinpoint the exact cause of back pain (Waddell and Turk 1992).

Elucidating the physical cause of pain is obviously important in acute pain, and every effort should be made to produce a cure when possible. In most cases, acute pain resolves with treatment or on its own within three months, although some recent studies suggest longer recovery times for back patients (for example, Von Korff and Saunders 1996). Typically, there's no need to uncover any nonphysical factors that may be influencing the pain. During the acute stage, physical factors dominate.

However, as pain progresses, physical factors take a backseat. Although physical factors still exert significant influence, research has consistently shown that your fears, your beliefs, and how you go about managing your pain are more important in explaining your suffering and disability and even, to some degree, the intensity of pain you experience (Turk and Monarch 2002). The further you are from the time of your injury or onset of pain, the more important the role of psychosocial factors in explaining why you hurt and how you cope with pain.

Addressing chronic pain requires your attention to the multiple layers of your pain problem. Approaches focused exclusively on a cure simply do not work. You need to manage your chronic pain, not try to cure it, and pay attention to the nonphysical factors that influence your pain experience.

I'll say more about acceptance of pain later in this book. For now, try to keep in mind that turning your attention to managing, rather than curing, your pain does not mean giving up the fight. People expend so much energy trying to eliminate their pain that their lives are put on hold waiting for the cure. Richard Sternbach, a well-known pain psychologist, wrote that if a number of reputable doctors have told you there's nothing more that can be done to cure your pain, accept it and move on (1983). The problem for many people is that they confound pain with suffering, believing that the only way out of their suffering is to eliminate their pain.

Pain, Suffering, and Disability

You may have been brought up to believe that pain, suffering, and disability are a package deal. However, nothing could be further from the truth.

Disability is what you cannot do that you once were able to do. It denotes a reduced ability to engage in activities and experience a wide range of behaviors, mood states, and thoughts as a result of a physically impairing condition, such as a herniated disc.

Suffering is the emotional side of pain, or what one fibromyalgia patient called "the awfulness" of pain. Pain triggers an emotional reaction for reasons of survival. When nociception (the physical cause of pain) is initiated, the emotional centers of the brain react negatively to motivate us to do whatever is necessary to reduce or avoid pain. If the emotional reaction weren't strongly negative, we wouldn't be as inclined to take action to protect ourselves.

Suffering is affected by nociception, but how you interpret your pain determines the level of suffering you experience. This is where things get complicated. If, for example, anytime you experience pain you worry that it may spin out of control and incapacitate you, your anxiety will increase as a consequence, amplifying your pain and suffering and fueling a vicious cycle.

There's a commonsense notion that if nociceptive input is high, disability and suffering will be correspondingly high. This is why most doctors view disability and suffering as simply incidental to the degree of physical impairment a person experiences. In reality, however, disability, suffering, and physical impairment are only weakly associated in people with chronic pain. Nonphysical factors have a huge influence on disability and suffering, and these factors are unique to each individual.

Disability is, in part, related to the physical cause of your pain. But what you can or cannot do is also connected to your fears of reinjury or being incapacitated by pain, and how you go about your day-to-day activities. Here are some of the factors most directly tied to disability level:

- Fears of pain or reinjury

- Physical deconditioning

- Fatigue

- The physical cause of pain

- A boom-and-bust approach to activities

- Adverse effects of medication

- The influence of others

- Unwillingness of the workplace to accommodate physical limitations

In a similar way, suffering is related to the physical problems you have. But the awfulness or misery you experience is also determined by what you expect will happen to you if you can't control your pain. Here are some of the factors most directly tied to level of suffering:

- The physical cause of pain

- Loss of income

- Reduction in pleasant activities

- Social isolation

- Fears that the pain will worsen

- Fears of physical incapacitation

- Fears of strained relationships or loss of relationships

- Fears of loss of productivity

- Fears of being incapacitated psychologically

Since suffering and disability are only modestly related to the physical aspects of pain, they can be modified without having to eliminate pain. This is a very optimistic message for you and others experiencing persistent pain.

■ Andy's Story

Andy's knee was severely damaged when a heavy industrial tire weighing over four hundred pounds tipped over, crushing his leg. He underwent several knee operations to repair the damage without any improvement in his pain. He finally had a total knee replacement, but the surgery caused extensive nerve damage, leaving him much worse off. He was treated with steroid injections, countless medications for pain relief, and physical therapy, but none of these provided him with significant long-term relief. Eventually Andy lost his job and had to declare bankruptcy. He spent much of his time on the couch staring at the TV, wondering where his life was headed and dreading the future. He desperately wanted to return to his former life.

More than one doctor told Andy that nothing more could be done to take away his pain, but he refused to accept this and thought it a death sentence of sorts. How could he ever have a decent quality of life in the presence of constant pain? He was convinced that as he aged his pain would inevitably worsen. He was depressed and suffering greatly.

It was only when Andy came to terms with his diagnosis that he started to engage in his life again. He turned his attention to why he was suffering and found that much of it had to do with his fears of failing in a new career, and the distress in his marriage caused by his financial problems. With the assistance of a counselor, he put together a vocational plan. Andy also learned better ways to cope with his pain, including living within his physical limitations, and he weaned himself from narcotics. He was able to start trucking school, and in a relatively short period of time he secured a job driving a truck locally. With this new job, his self-esteem improved and most other things in his life fell into place.

Andy still complains of pain, and every day he has to pay attention to things he learned from his psychologist about coping with pain better and keeping his mood upbeat. But his life is back in his control and he's suffering a lot less. He managed this not by eliminating his pain but by paying attention to making his life better in the presence of pain.

The Relationship Between Pain, Threat, and Anxiety

Like Andy, most people find that their suffering decreases when they change their perspective on the threats they had associated with pain. Indeed, a sense of threat is at the heart of why people suffer (Cassell 1982). When people expect bad things to happen, they suffer more, and when they believe things will work out, they suffer less.

When working with patients, I like to illustrate this concept by asking them to pretend the pen I'm holding is a magic wand. Then I ask them, "If I could promise I could take away your pain five minutes from now, would you suffer? You would have pain for those five minutes, but would you suffer?" Most reply, "If I believed my pain would go away after only five minutes, I'd be ecstatic. Anyone can deal with five minutes of pain." Although the example is admittedly far-fetched, it nicely illustrates the point that much of the misery people with chronic pain experience comes from expecting bad things to happen if they can't get rid of or significantly reduce their pain.

"My pain will increase as I age" is a common belief, as is "I've been so miserable since this started, how could things ever improve?" People often look at their increased limitations and other problems they attribute to pain and conclude that the underlying physical condition causing their pain has worsened. But in fact, as stated earlier, increased disability is often related to nonphysical factors, the primary exception being general deconditioning.

Closely tied to the sense of threat is a sense of vulnerability. When you believe you don't have the means to combat your pain, you suffer more because you can't imagine coping well. On the other hand, when you have confidence about wrestling with the multitude of problems that can occur as a consequence of pain (for example, financial loss, strain in relationships, or securing a new job), the sense of threat due to future loss diminishes, reducing suffering and changing the experience of pain. Depression, a common consequence of chronic pain, compounds the problem of suffering since a negative mood heightens a person's sense of vulnerability and fuels the belief that things will inevitably sour despite any efforts to change things.

ANXIETY AND AVOIDANCE

People with chronic pain report problems with anxiety and tend to be more fearful than the general population (Craig 1994). There are many explanations of why this is the case, but most experts believe that when people in pain develop negative expectations about physical harm or some other serious threat associated with pain, they avoid whatever they believe places them at risk. Avoidance may reduce the threat temporarily, but it reinforces the belief that something bad might have happened if the threat hadn't been avoided.

An elevated sense of threat is problematic in other ways, too. The emotional centers of the brain also pay more attention to and can amplify information considered threatening. In this way, your pain may increase even though from a purely physical standpoint your condition hasn't appreciably worsened. With acute pain, some avoidance makes good sense as it promotes healing, but in chronic pain, avoidance and other protective measures you take can reinforce your expectation of harm, fueling a vicious cycle.

HOW AVOIDANCE CAN WORSEN PAIN

A number of studies conducted in the past ten years show that a fear of pain can actually play a role in the maintenance of pain over time (Asmundson 1999). One study demonstrated that fear of pain is a strong predictor of disability, especially in terms of interference in daily activities (McCracken, Zayfert, and Gross 1993). Gorden Waddell, a famous Scottish orthopedist, discovered that pain-related fear is a strong predictor of work-related disability in low back pain patients (Waddell et al. 1993). When people believe their work might harm their back, they're much more likely to show higher levels of disability regardless of their physical condition. In fact, some studies indicate that a fear of pain is a stronger predictor of disability (for example, inability to return to work and low activity levels) than bio-medical indicators, such as the extent of physical impairment (Asmundson 1999).

It's important to understand that avoidance in response to the perceived threats associated with pain can involve much more than just how much you limit your physical activities. People with persistent pain also avoid by distracting themselves, taking pain pills or drinking to blunt anxious thoughts, con-stantly seeking reassurance even after it's been given, using walking aids when there's no need to, staying at home in antici-pation of flare-ups, and avoiding stressful situations out of con-cerns their pain may increase.

CHECKING BEHAVIORS

Many people with chronic pain also engage in behaviors designed to reassure themselves the pain isn't out of control. Called *checking behaviors*, these are more subtle forms of avoidance that involve engaging in activities that precipitate pain. Although this strategy is self-defeating, in the short run it provides reassurance that the person hasn't been defeated by pain, especially in regard to limitation of activities believed to signal a loss of function. For example, a patient named Debbie forced herself to vacuum the living room every day as she had before her injury, even though she knew it always caused her pain to flare up. She said she wasn't going to let the pain get the best of her and cripple her, as had happened to her mother after a failed hip operation.

CONFRONTING PAIN

Reducing the sense of threat associated with pain requires *gradually* confronting those things that trigger discomfort. This doesn't mean you should ignore your pain, charging ahead no matter what the consequences. This would cause an unending cycle of pain and validate the sense of threat that led to avoidance in the first place.

Confrontation is a balancing act that requires moving toward activities that might increase your pain, but doing so in a way that doesn't cause your pain to flare up. Constantly testing your limits by working to your pain tolerance will inevitably backfire—the boom-and-bust dynamic mentioned earlier. You need to respect your limitations while learning to move toward, not away from, activities in a way that doesn't reinforce fears of pain and its consequences.

Exercise: Understanding How a Sense of Threat Influences Your Pain

Take some time to think about what your pain means to you, and in what ways you find pain or its consequences threatening. Record your responses in your journal, and examine the different ways you avoid the threats associated with your pain. Ask yourself if you agree or disagree with the following statements. If any of the statements seem true to you, you may be experiencing a fear of pain.

- I need to restrict most of my activities until my pain is gone.

- I worry I might fall apart psychologically if I can't control my pain.

- I sometimes think that if I don't get rid of my pain, I could end up in a wheelchair.

- Physical activities that increase my pain could be harming me.

- The best way to cope with my pain is to limit my activities.

- I worry frequently that my pain may never go away.

- I can't stand the thought of not being able to eliminate my pain.

- Rest is best when it comes to controlling my pain.

- Pain and a decent quality of life are incompatible.

Mastering Personal Control

This book is all about mastering a stronger sense of personal control—a core skill in managing pain better and putting your life back in order. If you've been beaten down by the adversity of chronic pain, you can learn what to do to regain personal control and the belief that your future will be all right. You can learn to trust yourself as you face the difficulties of a life with chronic pain, and come to see that pain and a good quality of life aren't incompatible. This will help decrease the awfulness of pain and lessen the negativity associated with it.

This chapter has presented a great deal of information to help you understand the nature of chronic pain, suffering, and disability. Because this understanding is crucial for implementing the rest of this book's solutions, learning all of this background information truly is the first step in improving your situation. The foundation is laid, and now it's time to commit to real and significant behavior changes to help you better manage your pain and improve your quality of life. The remaining chapters will introduce you to techniques you can use to manage your pain by easing your suffering and disability. You'll be pleasantly surprised how simple and straightforward many of these techniques are.

2

Making Behavior Changes That Last

Changing behavior is tough. Even tougher, however, is sticking with the changes you make so that you can manage your pain better for a lifetime. This is a tall order no matter what approaches you decide to use, but not mission impossible if you set out on the right course from the beginning.

Is Willpower the Answer?

Most people believe that failure to change is due to a lack of willpower, as evidenced by the common expression "Where there's a will, there's a way." However, ask yourself what willpower is and how a person comes by the determination to take on difficult tasks such as stretching daily, learning how to relax, and pacing activities. Do you simply make your mind up to be serious once and for all?

Willpower is important for changing behavior, but it's not sprinkled onto us like fairy dust or granted to just a few lucky souls born with the right stuff. If you believe this, you're likely to sit and wait until the will to do something magically arrives to carry you to success. You might have to wait a very long time. Instead, think of willpower as something you create. By structuring things to stimulate your will, you can create the determination to do something. In other words, where there's a way, there's a will. This twist to the common expression carries important implications for any effort you decide to make to change your behavior so that you can manage your pain better. In essence, it means you can create the way by using strong incentives, changing your beliefs and behaviors, and adopting certain skills.

Consider the case of Charlotte, who wanted to start walking as part of her conditioning program. She made a commitment to walk very early in the morning, and she set an initial goal of two miles. Unfortunately, her plan was doomed from the start. Charlotte wasn't a morning person, and the most she had ever walked since her back injury was half a mile. After three days, she started looking for any and every excuse to avoid walking. She would have been more successful had she chosen to exercise during the day and set her initial goal at a quarter mile. She also could have made walking more fun and rewarding. Since Charlotte loves music, she might have used her husband's MP3 player when she walked. And instead of walking around the block, she could have driven two miles to the neighborhood park she loves to visit. Making her walks more fun and stimulating would have given her the will to succeed.

Maximizing Gains and Minimizing Costs

Above all else, creating the way requires that you maximize gains associated with your behavior change plan and minimize costs.

Make your efforts more rewarding and less punishing. A simple commitment to change isn't enough. Once stated it may seem obvious, but the reason for this is that you'll resist your efforts to change since what you're currently doing is more reinforcing than what you'd like to do—otherwise you wouldn't be doing what you're doing! It's human nature to engage in ingrained habits, despite sometimes negative consequences. A case in point is people who continue to smoke despite full knowledge of how cigarettes threaten their health. People use excuses and a fair dose of denial so that they can continue to smoke. Not until the costs outweigh the gains is the smoker motivated to change, such as when a doctor diagnoses emphysema. Only when individuals create a stronger way, making it more reinforcing to want to quit, is willpower stimulated.

Although change is difficult, you'll find it far easier and more rewarding if you keep a couple of strategies in mind. As each pain management solution is presented, ask yourself, "How can I create the way to help me succeed?" and "What can I do that will make it easier, more fun, and less odious?" Whenever you commit to making changes in behavior, consider how you can maximize your gains and minimize costs, keeping in mind these guidelines:

MAXIMIZING GAINS

- Follow your efforts with something rewarding (for example, TV or music).

- Draw up a contract or formal agreement with yourself to work toward specific goals.

- Use prompts, cues, or other simple reminders to trigger your behavior (for example, notes, pictures, or colored dots).

- Make your efforts fun. Be creative!

MINIMIZING COSTS

- Begin gradually, using small steps.

- Learn the skills presented in this book, which will help you change.

- Set goals that are within your reach and keep your overall expectations realistic.

- Practice your new habits at convenient times.

- Practice in convenient settings (for example, close to home).

- Set your initial goal at a level that guarantees your success.

People fail in their efforts to change for many reasons, but remember, beating yourself up and succumbing to guilt will only discourage you. Whenever you're stumped, go back to the drawing board and figure out a better way. Get rid of anything keeping you stuck in a rut and make it more rewarding to work toward goals you believe will help you feel better.

Exercise: Steps for Creating a Better Way

If you want your efforts to last more than a few days or weeks, you need to create a better way to learn how to stimulate your will. This exercise will guide you through a step-by-step process for effectively changing your behavior. As you work through the exercise, write your responses to the questions raised in your journal.

1. **Make a personal commitment to change.** To strengthen your commitment, look at your current lifestyle. Are you happy

with the way things are going? What would it mean to change your lifestyle to manage your pain better? Will things improve if you do nothing?

2. **Establish specific goals for change.** Vague goals such as "I want to feel better" are valid, but they don't provide you with any clear direction, and they're difficult to track. Goals such as "I want to walk ten minutes a day" and "I want to be able to sit without standing for thirty minutes" are more specific and useful. Try to choose specific goals from all of the following areas:

- **Physical**, such as improving your flexibility and strength

- **Activity**, such as increasing your pleasant activities

- **Mood**, such as reducing your depression, anger, and anxiety

- **Interpersonal**, such as improving communications with your spouse or other loved ones

- **Relaxation**, such as learning breathing techniques

- **Reducing use of medication** if not medically contraindicated

- **Reducing nonproductive beliefs,** such as catastrophic thinking (you'll learn more about nonproductive beliefs and catastrophic thinking in chapter 5)

3. **Prioritize your goals.** Some of your goals will take longer to achieve than others. At first, concentrate on goals that will increase your mobility and help reduce your sense of threats associated with pain. Activity-related goals are important first steps. Longer-term goals might include working on your self-esteem, returning to work, and gaining some of the strength you've lost.

4. **Minimize the costs associated with your behavior change plan.** Try to think how you can make your efforts to change your behavior less punishing. Not setting your goals too high is an example. Start slowly and set initial goals you can achieve. It's also important to remove other commitments that compete for your time and be sure to set aside enough time to implement your plan. Finally, examine any reservations you have about changing your lifestyle and try to figure out ways to overcome them.

5. **Maximize your gains.** Make change fun and rewarding. Use whatever incentives you can think of to stimulate and encourage your efforts. For example, if you reach your goal of doing your stretches a certain number of times each day, you can watch your favorite TV program. Rewards provide helpful positive reinforcement, but also use strategies that remind you to adhere to

your change program: notes, lists, and even colored dots placed in conspicuous places. Be creative and use whatever helps you get going and keep going. It's also important that you remove any competing reinforcers that might undermine your efforts to change. An example from a patient who was trying to lose weight is "Get the danger foods outta the house."

6. **Watch the excuses and denial.** Make a list of your excuses for not doing your stretches, not practicing your relaxation techniques, or not following through on any of your commitments. Remember, the pull is always back to your old habits. Excuses and denial ease the tension for failing to meet your goals. They also allow old habits to prevail. Here are some common excuses:

- I'm too stressed.

- I'm too tired.

- It doesn't matter anyway.

- I'm in too much pain.

- I'll wait until later, when my pain is better.

- If I try, I might make my pain worsen.

- These exercises may help others, but they won't help me.

7. **Never use guilt as a motivation for change.** If you fail to meet your goals, chalk it up as a sign that you need to go back to the drawing board and create a stronger way. Maybe your incentives for change weren't rewarding enough, or maybe your plan was too complicated. Don't attribute any failures to a lack of will and consider them signs of weakness; instead, simply rework your plan and start over.

8. **Prepare yourself mentally for change.** Look at your reasons for wanting to change and consider what you'll have to give up if you're successful. Even though you're in pain, are you settled in a lifestyle that you believe keeps you relatively comfortable or secure? Would change jeopardize the comfort and safety you think you have?

9. **Consider what change would mean to those around you.** Will those close to you support your efforts or try to undermine what you're doing? Do significant others in your life think of you as sick and disabled? What role, if any, do they play in your avoidance of certain activities and the way you manage and think about your pain? Can you gain their cooperation and support? Will change threaten them in any way?

In this chapter, you've learned how to develop an effective plan for behavior change by making a commitment to change, setting reasonable goals, and maximizing gains and minimizing costs. You can continue to refine your plan as you learn more, especially about the practical steps you can take to better manage your pain. Get in the practice of reworking your goals when you need to, and remember to be flexible in your approach. This chapter has emphasized that a successful plan depends on the right kinds of information, and to that end chapter 3 will help you demystify pain by taking charge and asking the right questions, laying a firm foundation for implementing changes to improve your quality of life.

3

Removing the Mystery of Pain

I f pain were a short-term disruption in your life, most of the information presented in this book would be unimportant. You would simply take your pills and sit tight, and the discomfort would eventually fade away. Unfortunately, this is not the case. You need all the good information you can get to help you develop the skills necessary to meet the challenges of living with pain. This chapter will help you understand why good information is so critical and how to get the right information to effectively manage your pain.

Pain is an undesirable experience that can leave you feeling stressed and out of control. Reestablishing personal control is important, but it's difficult to do so when you face the many uncertainties associated with chronic pain. It's particularly difficult to deal with the ambiguities of medical diagnoses and to confront a medical system that's frequently unresponsive to meeting the needs of patients, including the desire to know more.

■ Jeff's Story

Jeff was angry and frustrated. He injured his back when he slipped and fell, but he figured it was only a temporary problem. Days later, unable to get any relief from over-the-counter pain pills, he went to his family doctor, who told him his problem was a lumbar strain. He received a prescription for stronger anti-inflammatory medications and was referred to physical therapy, but after three weeks he still hadn't noticed any improvement. He scheduled a follow-up with his doctor, and his wife accompanied him to the visit. The doctor told Jeff to keep taking the medications but to quit the physical therapy since Jeff complained it was hurting him. The doctor performed an X-ray that was inconclusive but showed possible signs of degenerative disc disease.

When Jeff left the doctor's, he and his wife felt more confused and uncertain than they had before the appointment. Jeff had no idea what activities he could perform physically, what the normal course of back pain was, what treatments if any were available to him if he didn't respond to the medications, and what the next step in his care might be.

Seven months after his injury, Jeff was no better. He was referred to an orthopedic surgeon, who told him he had signs of an irritated sciatic nerve, but when he went to a neurosurgeon for a second opinion, the diagnosis and recommended treatment differed from what the orthopedist had said. He told both surgeons he wanted to avoid surgery and was referred back to his family doctor, who didn't have any suggestions other than a new prescription for stronger pain pills and to give physical therapy another try.

The new physical therapist worked for a rehabilitation center. He sat and listened to Jeff's concerns and the confusion he had about his back treatment, especially about how best to proceed. The therapist answered his questions, reviewed his medical chart in detail with him, and prescribed various exercises, accompanied by a detailed explanation of how the exercises would likely help him. He also gave Jeff material to read about the conservative treatment of back pain, and at each session he took time to review the materials he assigned and clarify any points of uncertainty. The therapist also spoke with Jeff's family doctor about this treatment approach.

When Jeff went to his next doctor's appointment, he had a list of questions for his doctor, and when he left he made sure that he and his doctor had a clear and specific game plan for managing his pain. Slowly, Jeff started to make improvements. His activity level increased, and he was able to cut down on his medications.

Remove Uncertainty with Information

The best medicine for Jeff was obtaining information that helped remove uncertainties about his back pain. Information is critical because when you're confused and uncertain, you lose your sense of personal control, increasing the sense of threat associated with your pain. The medical system often leaves patients out of the loop, floundering for direction and wondering what steps to take to facilitate recovery.

Jeff was fortunate. He had a physical therapist who educated him, and in a sense showed him the ropes. Managing pain is a lot more difficult than taking a ten-day course of antibiotics. You have to maneuver your way through a maze of decisions about which treatments are best with what doctors for what type of condition. You often must confront insurance companies who resist paying for treatments or restrict the kinds of care you receive. You may be left alone for weeks at a time between doctor's appointments, wondering what you should do and feeling hopeless and defeated by the health care system.

Take Charge

You need to take charge. Self-help books like this one can teach you specific techniques, but you need to do more. You need to let go of the idea that you're a passive participant with little control. Start asking questions, no matter how awkward you feel at first. Doctors and other health care providers don't know everything about pain, especially chronic pain, so keep your expectations realistic and approach your questions with a sense of fairness. Doctors want to see you get better, but they may not know the kind of information you need to help you move toward feeling less uncertain and more in control. Tell them what you need to know. Chapter 10 will provide an in-depth discussion of good communication with doctors and strategies you can use, so for now, just keep in mind that you have the right to know and that you can get the information you need with a little persistence.

In addition to books and other print materials, the Internet is an excellent source of information to help clear the air of confusion. Keep in mind, however, that you will sometimes come across inaccurate advice. Always seek the opinion of your doctor and other health care providers to verify the validity of information you find in your research. Also be aware that you'll probably read conflicting recommendations about the best way to manage pain, since much of what is known about chronic pain isn't grounded in years of controlled studies. This realm is an evolving science, so approach the advice you read with common sense and a healthy dose of skepticism.

Seek the Right Kind of Information

One of the most important purposes of gathering information is to help you move toward a greater sense of personal control to reduce the threats associated with pain. To that end, use the guidelines below to help you focus your search:

Guidelines for performing activities safely. Make sure your doctors and other health care providers outline the steps and strategies you can use to safely do different activities. You need to know what you can do safely and easily, and which activities require a more careful approach. Not knowing generates uncertainty, and as discussed, this breeds anxiety and the tendency to avoid. Make sure to ask for specific advice, such as how many minutes you can walk or what amount of weight you can lift. Recommendations such as "listen to your body" are too vague, and too focused on pain, which isn't useful when you have chronic pain.

Things you can do on your own to take care of your health. Ask for help in setting up a home program. Taking care of your health puts you in command and gives you a greater sense of mastery and control. You'll feel better when you believe you're doing more to help yourself. Sitting passively and waiting for things to be done to you throws you in the backseat. For example, a physical therapist should do more than just apply therapies to make you feel better (for example, massage); he or she should teach you techniques and exercises, such as safe stretches and lifting techniques, that you can take home and use to manage your pain better. Ask your physical therapist for a home program, and if he or she doesn't listen to you, find another therapist who will.

Potential consequences or side effects of treatments. Every treatment has a downside—there are no exceptions. If a doctor or other health care provider tells you a treatment is "perfectly safe," press for information about possible side effects and complications. Even stretching can cause problems if not done correctly. Your doctor can also help you understand what steps can be taken to avoid potential problems and side effects. Just because a potential problem is associated with a particular treatment doesn't necessarily mean you should refuse to give it a try. Sometimes you have to weigh the benefits against the costs. But if the costs outweigh the gains you're receiving or expect to receive, it's probably not the right treatment for you.

Whether the treatment is absolutely necessary. What is likely to happen if you opt against any given treatment? Ask your doctor to help you separate out which treatments are optional. Concerns about possible paralysis and other dire consequences due to refusing treatment should be taken very seriously, but rarely is refusing a particular treatment likely to result in something so dire. Get a second and even third opinion to reassure you and help you make the right decision.

The most realistic outcomes for particular treatment options. Inquire as to the percentage of people who improve greatly, moderately, and marginally and how many people experience a worsening of their condition with the recommended treatment.

Basic information about your legal rights. This is especially important if your injury is covered by workman's comp. This information can be gleaned from your insurance company, your employer, your state's division of insurance regulation, and some attorneys.

Information about your medical condition. Have someone knowledgeable sit down with you to explain your diagnosis and what exactly is known about your condition and what remains unclear. Don't hesitate to ask for an explanation of any terms you don't understand. Beyond your doctors, other good sources of information are nurses, pain psychologists, and physical and occupational therapists. Keep in mind that just because you have a diagnosis or results from imaging studies (such as an MRI) that indicate possible physical causes, such as a bulging disc, it doesn't necessarily mean you have serious cause for concern. A high percentage of adults who experience no pain show significant signs of pathology, including bulging discs. Ask your health care professionals whether your condition is dangerous—in the vast majority of cases it isn't. Only in rare cases are chronic pain problems catastrophic. It's likely that your medical problem is stable and relatively benign. Remember, hurt and harm are not necessarily the same in chronic pain.

Here's one last pointer on gathering information, especially from various health care practitioners: Remember, since knowledge about treatments for most pain conditions lacks solid scientific grounding, the advice you receive will be biased by the training of the specialist. Surgeons solve problems by cutting, and anesthesiologists are trained to use needles. Psychologists emphasize the psychology of pain, and physiatrists tend to look at pain problems from a musculoskeletal perspective. All perspectives have a kernel of truth, and no one perspective is the end-all in explaining the complexities of pain.

Exercise: Ask Your Doctor

This chapter emphasized the importance of acquiring the right kind of information to help you better understand and manage your pain. Now it's time to commit to seeking information. Write down at least three questions of particular importance to you about your pain problem. If necessary, read over the list of guidelines about the types of information to focus on. Take your list of questions to your doctor and ask each one. Make sure you get your questions answered before you leave the office. Then write the answers in your journal so that you can keep track of what you learned.

Exercise: Reexamine Your Goals

Once you've completed the previous exercise, use the information you learned to reexamine the goals you wrote down in the final exercise in chapter 2. Did your conversations with your health care providers give you any ideas for additional things you want to work on? Did you learn anything that indicates you should make adjustments to any of your previous goals?

Although demystifying your experience of pain is likely to be an ongoing process, hopefully the guidelines in this chapter have helped you make a strong start. In chapter 4, you'll learn more about factors affecting your pain and how to track your pain and disability. This information is critical for monitoring your progress and further refining your goals and plans for behavior change.

4

Tracking Your Progress

Keeping track of your pain is important. It will help you understand the factors influencing your pain and determine whether your behavior change plan is producing the kinds of changes you want. You could rely on guesswork and hunches, but following your progress more precisely will keep you from making poor decisions about what works best for you. And because this will help you notice changes that otherwise might be too subtle to detect, it will provide motivation that will help you adhere to your plan.

Functional Analysis

Begin jotting down your thoughts and impressions about your pain in your journal. This will help you make connections between your pain and your thoughts, feelings, and activities; for instance, you may start to see a pattern where your pain intensity increases when you feel stressed. Uncovering these sorts of relationships is called a *functional analysis*. It basically involves recording your pain rating, the situation that preceded your pain rating, and any other things you want to monitor (such as mood). Although a functional analysis can be very involved and complex, it's best to keep it simple. Its primary purpose is to give you some general impressions of factors that may be influencing your pain.

Exercise: Tracking Your Experience of Pain

A tracking table like the one in this exercise is just one method of monitoring your pain. Feel free to use other means of tracking if something else works better for you. Regardless of your approach, commit to a tracking period of at least three days and no more than seven days, and try to make notes four times a day.

Each time you record your observations, note the date and time of day. Rate your pain intensity first on a scale of 1 to 10, with 10 being the most severe. Next, record your mood on a scale of 1 to 10, with 10 being the worst mood possible and 1 being the best mood possible. In the Activity column, rate your prior activity (within one to two hours) as low, medium, or high. You might also briefly describe what type of activity you did. In the Thoughts column, note whether your thoughts were anxious (A), depressed (D), angry (ANG), neutral (N), and/or calm (C). Here's an example:

Date	Time	Pain Intensity	Mood	Activity	Thoughts
7/2/06	8:00 a.m.	8	8	high; cleaned up the kitchen	A, D, ANG; frustrated that simple things have become so difficult
7/2/06	12:00 noon	6	6	low; laid on the couch	D; feel useless, bored, and worried I won't accomplish anything
7/2/06	4:00 p.m.	8	8	medium; drove to the bank	A; worried about finances and my job situation
7/2/06	8:00 p.m.	7	9	low; laid on the couch	A, D, ANG; If I hurt this much after doing nothing, how can I ever have a normal life?

Exercise: Making Statements About Your Pain

At the end of your three- to seven-day tracking period, come up with some general statements about your pain and use this information to fine-tune your behavior change plan. Record your conclusions in your journal. At a minimum, try to answer the following questions:

- Did your pain worsen when your mood was more negative? For example, did your pain increase when you felt anxious or depressed? Did the reverse hold true? Did a better mood usually correspond with less pain?

- What was the relationship between your activity level and pain? What activities in particular triggered an increase in your pain?

- How did you rate your mood and what were your thoughts at times when your pain increased? Did your thoughts become more anxious and your mood more negative? Was there any theme to the content of your thoughts, such as discouragement about the future or fears your pain would never calm down?

- Did you notice any relationship between your pain and interactions with friends and family? For example, did your pain increase or decrease when you were with family members? (See chapter 10 for more information on how others influence the experience of pain and disability.)

- In general, how did you cope with pain? Did you rest, take pain medication, ask others for help, cry, or something else?

- When your pain was at its worst, how long did it last (for example, minutes, hours, or days)?

Exercise: Setting Behavior Change Goals

After you've tracked your pain and answered the questions above, generate several tentative goals you can use in your behavior change plan and record them in your journal. Here are a few examples to get you started:

- Reduce my negative mood.

- Reduce my fears of pain.

- Reduce my discouraging thoughts about the future.

- Alter my activities to reduce how often my pain flares up.

- Learn relaxation skills to reduce my anxious thoughts and negative mood.

- Change the way I interact with my family in regard to my pain.

In later chapters, you'll learn how to refine your goals to make them more meaningful and specific.

Keeping Track of Your Disability

In the introduction you learned about disability. As you may recall, disability refers to what you can't do that you used to be able to do before the onset of your pain. In addition to tracking your pain to determine how your pain is related to various factors, it's important that you also monitor your disability. This is because you want your behavior change plan to help you lower your disability. Lower levels of disability mean you're doing more, feeling better, and feeling less distressed about your pain.

Below is the Behavioral Assessment of Pain Screening Instrument, or BAPSI, a simple rating of disability. Use the BAPSI to periodically assess how you're doing (for example, once per week). Examine your high scores (5, 6, 7) since they may give you additional clues for targets you may want to focus on in your behavior change plan. Record your BAPSI scores in your journal.

Exercise: The BAPSI Questionnaire

The following survey examines how your pain has changed your life. For each statement below, select the one answer that best describes how much you agree or disagree with the statement.

For example, if you strongly agree with an item, answer 5, 6, or 7. If you strongly disagree with an item, answer 0, 1, or 2. If you moderately agree or feel neutral about an item, answer 3 or 4.

0	1	2	3	4	5	6	7
Strongly disagree					Strongly agree		

1. I'm not as physically strong as I used to be before developing pain. _____

2. I avoid situations that might make my pain worse. _____

3. I don't have as much energy as I used to before developing pain. _____

4. I don't sleep as well as I used to before developing pain. _____

5. I take prescription pain medication daily. _____

6. I'm not as physically active as I used to be before developing pain. _____

7. I've felt stressed during the past week. _____

8. I've gone to the emergency room in the past six weeks because of my pain. _____

9. I've been off work more than six weeks because of my pain. _____

10. I've lost interest in many activities I used to enjoy. _____

11. I'm having difficulty taking care of my responsibilities because of my pain. _____

12. I find it difficult to motivate myself to do things. _____

13. I use alcohol to cope with my pain. _____

14. I've expressed feelings of sadness and depression during the past week. _____

15. My sex life isn't as satisfying as it used to be. _____

16. My pain has caused problems in my marriage or relationship. _____

17. I've visited a doctor, chiropractor, or physical therapist more than ten times in the past month because of my pain. _____

18. Over the past week, I've felt useless and inadequate. _____

19. My pain problem is more than I can handle. _____

20. I worry about reinjuring myself. _____

21. I've felt irritable during the past week. _____

22. I'm not able to work as well as I used to before developing pain. _____

23. I can't do my chores around the house as well as I used to before developing pain. _____

Add up the points for all twenty-three items. Use the following scoring criteria as a general guide, but don't concern yourself too much with the severity level (severe, moderate to severe, and so on). Instead, focus more on the change in point value from week to week:

130 or more	Severe
100 to 129	Moderate to severe
70 to 99	Moderate
40 to 69	Mild to moderate
39 or less	Mild

For a more precise scoring of the BAPSI, you can go to my Web site HealthNetSolutions .com, where, for a nominal fee, you can take the BAPSI online. The printout will produce a disability index score and a psychological distress score. Whether you complete the questionnaire in this book or online, share the results with your doctor and other health care providers, and record your results in your journal so you can compare from week to week.

Tracking your pain and performing a functional analysis will help you see patterns in how your pain intensity relates to your mood, activities, and thoughts. Armed with this knowledge, you can fine-tune your goals and develop more effective behavior change programs. To further enhance your ability to manage your pain and reduce your disability, it's crucial to learn to recognize, understand, and change other, more subtle patterns: patterns of nonproductive thinking. The next chapter focuses on this important skill.

5

Changing Your Nonproductive Beliefs

This chapter concerns your beliefs about your pain. Research into this topic has clearly shown that when people adopt nonproductive beliefs about their pain experience, levels of disability and suffering increase, mood deteriorates, and pain intensity worsens. For example, people who interpret their pain as a result of ongoing tissue damage express more disability and experience higher levels of suffering than people who view their pain as a stable medical problem (Spiegel and Bloom 1983). Moreover, chronic pain patients require less medication when they believe the cause of their pain is relatively benign but they require considerably more pain medication when they think their pain is due to cancer (Cassell 1982). A series of studies also showed that a patient's performance on a number of physical activities was more related to beliefs of anticipated pain than to their actual pain ratings or physical exertion (Schmidt 1985a, 1985b).

When people believe their pain is an unexplainable mystery, they tend to downgrade their own coping abilities (Williams and Keefe 1991); they also tend to believe they have little or no control over their pain. This may relate to unsuccessful efforts to manage pain (Turk and Monarch 2002). Repeated failures to control pain can lead to the expectation of uncontrollable pain and can heighten the intensity of pain (Leventhal and Everhart 1979). If you believe you can't control your pain or prevent other problems from occurring, you're less likely to want to attempt being active. This can cause you to feel helpless and oversensitive to even slight increases in discomfort. Beliefs of controllability have been shown to be more highly related to tendencies to avoid activities than a person's actual physical status (Turk and Monarch 2002).

■ Bob's Story

Bob, a fifty-two-year-old car salesman, injured his back while lifting. After being off work for four months, he tried to return to his job, but with no success because the long hours of standing caused him too much pain. Bob was taking narcotic analgesics for his pain and seeing a physical therapist three times a week, mostly doing stretching exercises. After complaining to his doctor that he felt worthless, he was referred to me for an evaluation.

The thing that struck me most about Bob was his conviction that as long as he had pain he would never be happy. He felt that pain had ruined his life and that he had to get rid of it before he could return to his former self. He often worried that his doctors had given up on him and the physical therapist was just going through the motions, not really convinced he would respond to treatment. Bob also believed he had no control over his pain, especially since his doctors couldn't explain exactly why he hurt. Bob felt that his pain was a mystery and no one had the

skill to stop what he described as a runaway train.
Bob's convictions were so strong that they were
affecting his mood and his interpretation of his pain,
and these, in turn, were contributing to his inability
to resume more normal levels of activity.

How Thoughts and Beliefs Influence Pain, Disability, and Suffering

Clearly, beliefs exert a powerful influence on many aspects of the pain experience, most likely by affecting mood, elevating negative expectations and a sense of threat, and increasing physiologic arousal, especially levels of muscle tension. Additionally, the way people process information about their pain may cause a heightened awareness and preoccupation with bodily sensations, such as pain (Turk and Monarch 2002).

Bob believed his pain was incompatible with a good quality of life, and that as long as he had pain he would never be happy and could lose everything. His beliefs heightened his fears of pain, motivating him to avoid most activities. He was convinced that resuming his activities might risk making matters worse and prevent his recovery. Since Bob thought his pain was such a mystery, he felt uncertain about what he could do safely. The best way to cope, he surmised, was to lay low and wait. However, his beliefs were preventing him from doing what he needed to do to get better. If Bob didn't see a catastrophe brewing with every flare-up of his pain, or if he was able to more realistically examine the consequences of his pain, the threat he attributed to his pain would lessen. Understanding the underlying nature of his pain in more benign terms, rather than considering his bulging disc to be a disaster in waiting, would have allowed Bob to more realistically assess fearful concerns and begin to resume his activities.

The Origin of Nonproductive Beliefs

Nonproductive beliefs probably take hold in people with chronic pain because they're misinformed about their pain. If you've been told that dire consequences can occur if you're active, you'll probably believe that rest is safer than being active. If you limit your activities and experience a temporary reprieve from pain, the belief that inactivity is protective will be strengthened.

Early learning experiences can also contribute to the formation of nonproductive beliefs. This is particularly true with assumptions about control. When people's experiences have taught them that control and predictability are paramount for emotional well-being, they're likely to perceive the experience of chronic pain as considerably more threatening.

Bob described himself as a perfectionist. He liked his life structured, and he worked hard to keep things "steady state," as he put it. When I first met with Bob, he revealed that when he was in his early twenties, he was a mess—out of work, drinking too much, and always getting into some kind of trouble. One night he and a friend stopped off at a bar to have a drink. A man sitting next to him was drunk and kept bumping into Bob, spilling his drink on him. Although Bob tried to ignore him, the situation escalated until Bob punched the man so hard he knocked him unconscious. Bob fled from the bar but was later arrested and charged with battery.

This incident changed Bob's life. He stopped drinking and turned all his energies to keeping his nose clean. He worked excessive hours and never missed a day of work. Bob said it was important to prove to himself and others that he was a good person. This also meant keeping his emotions in check for fear he might revert to his former "bad" self.

After Bob's back injury, he did everything he could to regain his health. Unfortunately, his recovery was marred by numerous setbacks and the ups and downs of dealing with a workman's comp system that frustrated him at every turn with unnecessary delays and treatment denials for recommended care. He soon became depressed and anxious. He felt out of control and started to worry he would unravel both physically and psychologically. He started to imagine the worst and was worried he was slipping back into his old ways.

Fearing a loss of control is common among people with chronic pain. But because of Bob's past and how he'd struggled to cope by means of rigidity and perfectionism, this loss of control was much more threatening for him.

Another way to understand how early learning experiences can contribute to the formation of nonproductive beliefs is to think of pain as a threat associated with potential loss. If you believe you can meet the challenges of pain, you're less likely to adopt beliefs that disaster is imminent. This confidence about overcoming adversity is likely the result of positive past experiences that taught you you're capable of overcoming problems. However, if past experiences haven't inspired confidence, feelings of vulnerability will prevail, causing you to fear the threats associated with pain. Beliefs that losses are likely won't be easily dismissed and could take hold.

The Importance of Corrective Feedback

How do nonproductive beliefs persist when clearly they can aggravate and complicate the experience of pain and lead to greater levels of disability and negative mood? The main reason is that the person in pain minimizes experiences that would refute the validity of these beliefs. In other words, there's no corrective feedback (Turk and Monarch 2002). If, for example, you believe that certain activities are likely to cause you reinjury or a significant exacerbation of your pain, you will be discouraged from doing activities that would prove your assumptions incorrect. Your avoidance reinforces the negative expectation that something bad might have happened if you had done those activities. Fortunately, there are effective strategies for overcoming this dynamic, and in chapter 6 you'll learn the best way to overcome these thoughts: actively engaging in experiences that challenge and refute your nonproductive beliefs.

Types of Nonproductive Beliefs

Although there are many types of nonproductive beliefs, I've found that most nonproductive beliefs associated with chronic pain fall into four broad categories:

1. Beliefs about threatening outcomes

2. Beliefs of powerlessness

3. Overestimation of personal responsibility

4. Despair about the future

Let's take a closer look at these four types of beliefs and try to identify nonproductive thoughts that may be interfering with your ability to manage your pain.

BELIEFS ABOUT THREATENING OUTCOMES

Threatening beliefs are thoughts that spell doom and gloom associated with the experience of pain. They're highly charged with anxiety and often relate to fears of incapacitation and other dire outcomes if pain persists. They're often marked by a tendency to *catastrophize*, or expect the worst possible outcome.

Threatening beliefs can be organized into two categories: over-estimating probabilities and overestimating the severity of consequences (Antony and McCabe 2004).

OVERESTIMATING PROBABILITIES

People with chronic pain often predict events that are very unlikely. These thoughts may have a grain of truth to them, but are very unlikely to happen, and certainly not to the degree predicted. Expecting the worst is more likely when you feel vulnerable and unable to face the challenges you believe the pain might cause. Here are common thoughts that reflect an overestimation of probabilities:

- I'll fall apart psychologically if I don't control my pain.

- My spouse will leave me if I don't get rid of my pain.

- I'll never enjoy life again as long as I have pain.

- I worry I could end up in a wheelchair.

- I'm falling apart physically and will never be healthy again.

- As I grow older, my pain will inevitably worsen and the problems I'm having will double, maybe even triple.

- I feel so bad at times that I know the pain will cause an early death.

- If I don't control my pain, it will trigger my anxiety and I might suffocate, or even die.

- If I don't keep myself active day to day, the pain will overwhelm me.

- Getting rid of my pain is the most important thing I can do, because if I don't I'll lose my job and never find another one.

In general, most of these statements are completely untrue, and others are exaggerations that are very unlikely to occur. For example, being disabled by pain can be serious and can put a strain on your relationship, but this doesn't mean your marriage is likely to fail if your pain persists. Overestimating the catastrophic consequences of your pain doesn't help you in any way; rather, it leaves you feeling overwhelmed and anxious. Tempering your thoughts so that they're more realistic and grounded in fact can help you move forward and tackle the things you need to do to feel better.

Exercise: Identifying Overestimation of Probability

The following questions will help you identify any thoughts you have that reflect an overestimation of probability. Record your answers in your journal:

- What kinds of things are you most concerned about in regard to your pain?

- Do you have solid facts to support your concerns?

- What effects do your thoughts have on how you cope with your pain?

- If your thoughts weren't so exaggerated, would you attempt to do more things?

OVERESTIMATING THE SEVERITY OF CONSEQUENCES

Overestimating the severity of consequences involves concluding a particular outcome would be much worse than it really would be (Antony and McCabe 2004). It entails exaggerating the importance of your predictions. Here are some examples of beliefs that show an overestimation of consequences:

- If my doctors can't find something wrong with me, it would mean that there's something terribly wrong.

- If I have a pain flare-up at work, it would be a disaster since I wouldn't be able to do anything.

- If I have a pain flare-up, it could take months to calm down or it might never stop, for that matter.

- If my pain were to flare up severely, there's absolutely nothing I could do to cope.

- If my pain worsens, my family will suffer terribly.

- If my pain never goes away, it would mean I could never do the things that make life worthwhile.

- If my muscles spasm, I'll never be able to calm them down.

Overestimating the severity of consequences can have the same effect as overestimating probabilities. If you imagine that dreadful consequences will follow some event or activity, you'll be more likely to avoid the things you believe will lead to that outcome.

Exercise: Identifying Overestimation of the Severity of Consequences

Think about what you say to yourself when your pain flares up or when you imagine certain bad things occurring because of your pain. Do you have a tendency to overestimate the severity of the consequences? Answer each of the questions below and record your answers in your journal.

- What is the likelihood that the consequences you imagine will come true?

- What solid evidence do you have that if the event happens, the consequences you imagine happening will also occur?

- Has your doctor or other health care provider told you the consequences you imagine will actually happen?

BELIEFS OF POWERLESSNESS

The second category of nonproductive thoughts is beliefs of powerlessness—beliefs that you don't have the personal resources or ability to overcome the problems caused by pain. Here are some examples:

- I have no control over my pain.

- Without my medications, there's nothing I can do to manage my pain.

- I'm helpless in the face of my pain.

Chronic pain can be overwhelming. You might have thought, "I don't know how to deal with all the problems I'm up against." When you believe you can't cope when confronted with pain, you're much more likely to feel distressed, anxious, and depressed, and this holds true regardless of the severity of your physical problems.

It's no wonder you might not feel up to meeting the challenges of chronic pain, which involves so many things that are probably new and removed from your everyday experiences. Trying to understand the complexities of the medical system, for example, can be a daunting experience. However, when your thoughts reflect an exaggerated loss of confidence about being able to meet the challenges of chronic pain, the task of coping becomes more difficult.

Exercise: Understanding Your Beliefs of Powerlessness

Think about your pain and the problems you face every day with pain. Do you believe there's absolutely nothing you can do to cope? When pain gets you down, it's easier to focus on what you can't do and the numerous failures you've experienced. Instead, try to think of some of your successes no matter how insignificant you think they are. List your successes in your journal and use these to challenge unrealistic beliefs that you're powerless. Consider adding to the list of your successes periodically and reading over it any time you need a boost in your confidence.

OVERESTIMATION OF PERSONAL RESPONSIBILITY

At one time or another you've probably thought, "Could I be doing more to manage my pain or get better?" You also might have blamed yourself for events that precipitated your pain. Here are some examples of overestimating personal responsibility:

• I shouldn't have let myself get injured.

• I should be doing more to manage my pain.

• There must be something I'm doing wrong since I continue to hurt so much.

Most people with pain have these kinds of thoughts occasionally, but for some they occur often, even to the point of causing frequent feelings of guilt and depression. The underlying assumption driving these beliefs is that you should be able to control your pain, and maybe that you could have prevented it from occurring in the first place.

These kinds of beliefs are problematic because they overestimate your personal responsibility. Taking responsibility for managing your pain is good, but only when you know where you're headed and have developed the right skills for coping successfully with pain. Beating yourself up for failing to do more when confronted with the complexities of pain is unrealistic and unfair to you.

Exercise: Understanding Your Overestimation of Personal Responsibility

Take a few minutes to think about whether you're overestimating your personal responsibility. Consider the questions below and try to be realistic and fair with yourself. Write your responses in your journal.

- What more could you realistically be doing to better manage your pain?

- How did you fail to prevent your pain from occurring in the first place? What more could you have done? Are you being fair with your conclusions?

- Do you expect to always keep your pain under control? Is this realistic? If you did everything just right all the time, could you honestly expect to prevent any future flare-ups?

DESPAIR ABOUT THE FUTURE

The final category of nonproductive beliefs common to people with chronic pain involves despair about the future. It isn't uncommon to feel discouraged from time to time when confronted with the uncertainties and ups and downs of pain. You may have stopped trusting that the future will turn out okay and instead imagine that things will either stay the same or, worse, fall apart. Here are some examples of this type of thinking:

- The future is hopeless.

- My pain will only get worse as I age.

- Since things haven't worked out so far, they're unlikely to ever get better.

Exercise: Understanding Your Despair About the Future

What are your thoughts about the future? Do you get discouraged frequently and imagine only the worst possible outcomes? What medical proof do you have that your pain will worsen or that you won't cope well eventually? Write your thoughts in your journal.

Identifying Automatic Thoughts

By now you should have a better idea of the kinds of nonproductive beliefs that are particularly troublesome to you. The examples in the exercises above were designed to stimulate your thinking. However, nonproductive beliefs are often based on thoughts that are so habitual and ingrained that you may not be aware of them. Known as *automatic thoughts*, these thoughts are emotionally charged and based on faulty and unrealistic assumptions, such as "I will never be happy as long as I have pain." They occur repetitively and are often so fleeting you may only notice the anxiety, anger, or depression that follows their occurrence. If you sometimes feel emotionally upset but can't pinpoint any specific reasons why, it may be that automatic thoughts are involved. The next exercise will help you start to tune in to your automatic thoughts.

Changing Nonproductive Beliefs

Nonproductive beliefs are like stubborn habits. The good news is that you can change the way you think, but it takes dedication and practice. The more time you spend challenging your nonproductive beliefs, the better you'll become at refuting them.

At first, you may struggle with thinking more productively, and you might even dismiss the exercises as futile. If so, it's probably because even though the beliefs are getting you into trouble emotionally and adding to your disability, they somehow make sense of the world around you. You may even think they're keeping you safe or preventing a worsening of your condition. This, too, is something you need to examine. Are your nonproductive beliefs really keeping you from harm's way and protecting you from some imagined calamity? If your thoughts were less extreme, more realistic, and even more forgiving of your faults, would you feel differently? Would you be able to see the world in a more positive light and with much less anxiety?

THE TWO-STEP PROCESS FOR CHANGING NONPRODUCTIVE BELIEFS

Changing the automatic thoughts that underlie your nonproductive beliefs is a two-step process. The first step is to examine and challenge the evidence supporting your beliefs. The second step involves conducting behavioral experiments to help debunk false or extreme beliefs. This very powerful method of deciding if your beliefs are true involves playing the role of the scientist to discover what is most truthful (Antony and McCabe 2004).

STEP ONE: EXAMINE THE EVIDENCE

We often gravitate toward beliefs without examining the evidence that supports our thinking. Learning to question the cognitive errors underlying your nonproductive beliefs—faulty logic, erroneous assumptions, and exaggerated predictions—is at the heart of changing these beliefs. For example, the belief "I'll never be happy as long as I have pain" is faulty because it involves predicting the future—an impossible feat—and it's also based on an incorrect assumption. Just because someone has been unhappy and in pain doesn't mean they'll never be happy in the future. People with chronic pain can indeed be happy, especially after learning better ways of coping.

Examining the evidence essentially means scrutinizing the information you're using to support your beliefs. Is that information accurate? Did you check it against any available facts? Consider the belief "I'm likely to reinjure myself if I start a lifting program." Is this a known medical fact? What is it based on? Does this apply to all lifting? When you look at the likelihood of your predictions coming true, consider whether it's 100 percent. Might it be less, possibly a great deal less?

Oftentimes people in pain confuse feelings with facts to support their beliefs. An example would be "I'm likely to reinjure myself; my anxious feelings are warning me it could happen." However, feeling anxious isn't evidence that reinjury is likely. What specific evidence or facts support the thought that you're susceptible to reinjury?

Try to think of alternatives to your usual conclusions. Can you come up with possibilities other than those you tend to fall back on, sometimes automatically? For example, "I can't do anything to control my pain" could be reinterpreted as "I can usually do something to ease the pain, such as relaxing, taking a hot shower, or stretching."

Exercise: Weighing the Evidence

This exercise will help you challenge the non-productive beliefs you've written in your journal. For each nonproductive belief, use the format below to examine the evidence for and against the belief, then weigh the evidence. This process will help you identify more accurate and realistic ways of thinking. Here's an example:

Belief: *My pain will never settle down.*

Evidence that this is true: *I've heard stories of people having such high pain there was nothing they could do to bring it down.*

Evidence that this isn't true: *(1) My pain may increase at times, but it always settles down eventually. (2) Although I've heard stories of people having uncontrolled pain, I've never spoken to anyone who can verify this. (3) There's no known medical fact or anything my doctors have said to support the idea that my pain will never settle down.*

Weigh the evidence: *On the whole, there's no evidence my pain will never settle down. This is mostly something I feared, and I was interpreting my feelings as fact.*

Repeat this exercise daily for one week and then every other day for another week. After this, continue to do the exercise at least weekly to see if you still show a tendency to fall back on certain beliefs. If so, shorten your list and practice challenging those more stubborn beliefs.

STEP TWO: CONDUCT BEHAVIORAL EXPERIMENTS

One of the most powerful methods of challenging non-productive beliefs is to disprove them by conducting behavioral experiments (Greenberger and Padesky 1990). Weighing the evidence is critical in helping you begin to refute your troublesome beliefs, but people often develop such habitual ways of thinking that this purely intellectual exercise isn't enough. Behavioral experiments help you dispel beliefs by creating events to test whether your beliefs are true or not. You can't apply this technique to all of your nonproductive beliefs, but for most you can design experiments to refute your dire predictions and negative expectations (Antony and McCabe 2004).

The first step is to choose the nonproductive belief you want to test. Ask yourself what would happen if the belief were true and what would happen if it weren't. Next, set up an experiment to test your predictions. For example, let's look at the belief "If I walk on the treadmill for three minutes, I'll experience a pain intensity of 10." To test this belief, you'd go ahead and walk on the treadmill (assuming it's not medically contraindicated). You'd rate your pain before you walk on the treadmill and then again afterward to see if your pain flares up as much as you expected.

Here are some other examples you can use to help you devise effective experiments:

Nonproductive belief: If I don't constantly distract myself from my pain, it will increase and overwhelm me.

Experiment: Focus on your pain. Try to increase it by concentrating on it.

Nonproductive belief: If I don't have a pain pill before I run my errands, my pain will escalate out of control.

Experiment: Don't take a pain pill before you run errands. If you take pain pills regularly, schedule a trip to run errands sometime other than right after taking the medication.

Nonproductive belief: If I join my family for dinner when my pain is above average, everyone will have a miserable time, especially me.

Experiment: Have dinner with your family no matter how you feel. Stand or take a brief break if you need to.

Before you attempt any activity, however, make sure you're well within the guidelines established by your physical therapist or physician. If you haven't been given any guidelines, if you have but they're vague, or if you think they're too restrictive or too liberal, ask for clarification and a discussion of your concerns.

The Role of Acceptance

Acceptance of pain is important because it reflects a successful evolution in the way you think about your pain. Whereas fighting to get rid of *acute* pain makes sense, the situation with chronic pain is different. When nothing has helped and you've tried and tried but still have pain, sometimes it's good to let go.

For most people in chronic pain, this is one of the hardest things to do. Initially, it may seem that acceptance means giving up hope of ever feeling happy again. Nobody wants to resign themselves to chronic pain. It goes against human nature. The emotional brain is wired to fight or flee, not to let go and accept, especially when the consequences seem fearsome or threatening.

But consider what happens when you constantly push pain away and fight it with therapies that give you little or no relief. You never come to realize that the suffering you imagined might engulf and possibly destroy you doesn't occur. Pain is uncomfortable and nobody wants to live in constant pain, but pushing it away amplifies its importance and its intensity. With acceptance comes the realization that pain can be a part of your life without destroying what you believe makes life worthwhile.

Exercise: Thinking More Critically About Acceptance

Take some time to think about what acceptance means to you. What would it be like to live with pain for the rest of your life? If you stopped fighting the pain, would it destroy you? If you weren't constantly struggling to rid yourself of your pain, how could you turn your attention and energies to making your life better despite your pain? Write your responses in your journal. This exercise should help you identify more nonproductive beliefs about your pain. Write them down and challenge them by weighing the evidence.

Challenging your nonproductive beliefs is critical. The exercises you did in this chapter helped you identify those beliefs and replace them with more realistic thoughts. In the process, you've begun to control the distress caused by faulty thinking and experimented with doing things you feared. This is important, because activity is one of the keys to your ultimate success. The next chapter discusses ways of guaranteeing your success in increasing your activity level.

6

Being Active, Not Passive

P ain is naturally limiting. When we hurt, we want to rest and avoid those activities we believe aggravate our discomfort. As discussed earlier, this response to pain is adaptive with acute pain, since it can assist in the healing process. With chronic pain, however, too much avoidance of activity can cause health problems, such as muscle atrophy. Inactivity can also lead to diminished quality of life and negative mood, and as you've learned, avoidance can strengthen fears of pain, leading to an increase in discomfort and suffering.

The Boom-and-Bust Dynamic

Most people with chronic pain regulate their activity by pushing until they're in pain on good days, then doing nothing until they feel better, then repeating the process all over again. This boom-and-bust strategy doesn't work since it sensitizes you to be wary of pain, strengthening the belief that pain leads to bad consequences. It can also cause too much downtime as you recuperate. Increased avoidance of activity is the inevitable consequence of overdoing it.

If the strategy of overdoing things and working until you're in pain doesn't work, why do it? Because in the short run it works: some things do get accomplished and you experience a small victory because pain hasn't won the day. But the downside is guilt, more physical discomfort, and increased feelings of defeat and fears of pain in the long run.

As you become increasingly cautious and careful, more and more activities become triggers for pain. This is in part related to the general deconditioning that occurs with avoidance of activity. But it also happens because repeated flare-ups condition you to expect negative consequences from activity. This can become a vicious cycle as ever more activities become associated with pain, in turn leading to higher levels of avoidance.

■ Peggy's Story

Peggy, a twenty-four-year-old graduate student, had neck and shoulder pain caused by a car accident. She tried everything but surgery to eliminate her pain but without success. Physical therapy gave her the best relief, particularly the stretching techniques she learned.

In the three years since her accident, Peggy reduced her activities by more than 75 percent. She went to school every day but did little else. Riding in a car caused her the most discomfort. At first she charged ahead, forcing herself to be active at the insistence of her doctor. She knew it was important to remain active, but after experiencing nearly daily flare-ups in her pain, she began to cut back on things she worried would trigger her pain.

She tried to follow her physical therapist's advice to pace her activities, but to Peggy that meant slowing down and being more sensitive to when her pain started to increase. However, as she later learned, pacing doesn't necessarily require slowing the pace of activities or an increased sensitivity to the onset of increased pain.

A Balancing Act

Although you now understand the importance of activity, it's likely that your attempts to increase your activity have failed in the past. You've probably tried to fight your pain, avoided certain activities, taken extra medication when you were more active, pushed yourself only on good days, and slowed down so much on bad days that you accomplish very little. If you're ready to try something different, read on. This chapter will help you achieve success in increasing your activity level by helping you develop a pacing program.

As you begin to increase your activity level, it's important to take a gradual approach and not overdo it. It's a balancing act with certain important rules attached. It doesn't mean being tougher or fighting the pain—this never works. It does mean being smarter and using common sense and a systematic approach. In essence, pacing requires that you move away from the habit of working to the point of pain and instead work to reasonable quotas that are within your limitations. This doesn't mean you'll experience no discomfort, especially as you begin your pacing program. You'll have to confront your fears of pain and overcome the initial soreness and stiffness as you start to use atrophied muscles. However, by following the steps below you will succeed, no matter how discouraged you may feel.

ERRORLESS LEARNING

One story I like to tell to set the stage for introducing pacing involves basketball. In the early 1980s, the University of Houston, my undergraduate alma mater, had one of the best college teams. They made it to the championship game but lost by one basket as the buzzer sounded. Houston had a great team, but they had one weakness: a terrible free throw percentage. I like to speculate that if they'd been better at making free throw shots, they might have won the championship.

When I ask patients to imagine how they'd go about increasing Houston's free throw percentage, most respond by telling me they'd make the team practice free throw shots over and over. Although this is a good idea, it's probably something the coaches tried without success. When I ask patients to think outside the box, someone usually says, "I'd move the free throw line up right under the hoop." Exactly. You could even drop the hoop down a bit. As the player succeeds in meeting a minimal criteria during practice, say 80 percent, you would gradually raise the hoop and increase the distance. If at any point the player doesn't reach the 80 percent criteria, you'd go back to the previous step and only advance after the player achieved 80 percent again.

This technique, called *errorless learning*, can be used in pacing to help achieve increased activity levels. The basic idea is to adapt the desired behavior to a minimally demanding level in order to guarantee success—hence the name "errorless learning." Another way to think about the process is to use the analogy of a ladder. Start with the lowest rung to achieve success and move up from there.

Errorless learning is an important strategy to incorporate in your pacing program for three important reasons. First, it requires that you quit trying to meet unrealistic expectations. When patients tell me they can't lift anything, I hand them my pen. After a look of "Oh, come on," I tell them, "You said anything. If we have to start with a pen, then so be it. Let's find the level that's somewhat uncomfortable and move up from there." People with chronic pain need to experience success, not more failure and defeat. Making things simple and setting realistic goals helps assure that you have a positive outcome.

The second benefit to errorless learning is that it gradually reconditions you. Since chronic pain is associated with muscle atrophy, gradually increasing how much you do simply makes good common sense. The third and most important aspect of errorless learning is that it allows you to confront your fears of pain, movement, increased activity, and uncomfortable sensations in a stepwise fashion. Charging forward doesn't work. It only increases the likelihood of a flare-up, sensitizing you to pain. Although flare-ups are rarely associated with harm, it's hard to rationalize away concerns about your pain when you hurt so much.

GRADED EXPOSURE

Before we get into the specific steps to pacing, there's one more background issue to cover. If your pacing program is to succeed, it must incorporate strategies for reducing your fears. Errorless learning can help here, too, by allowing you to gradually and safely confront your fears of increased activity. With gradually increasing activity, you'll refute the negative expectation that something bad might happen because you're more active. This will reduce your fears and increase your confidence about doing more.

To guarantee your success, however, you need to expose yourself to all of the fears associated with your pain, not just increased levels of activity. The pacing techniques will encourage you to confront most of your activity-related concerns, such as fears of reinjury when lifting or bending at the waist, but unless you include the full spectrum of your fears, you'll continue to experience problems and be susceptible to activity avoidance.

Identifying your fears and systematically exposing yourself to them helps reduce your concerns and will make you more comfortable engaging in activities. Uncovering the specific fears associated with your pain isn't always easy, but your pain tracking and the techniques in this chapter should give you some good ideas of where to start.

STEPS IN DEVELOPING YOUR PACING PROGRAM

It's time to design your pacing program. The following steps, discussed in detail below, will help you plan your program:

1. Identify activities you avoid.

2. Establish baselines.

3. Develop an activity hierarchy.

4. Set your initial quotas.

5. Set your target goal.

6. Determine the rate of activity increase.

7. Log your activities daily.

8. Identify and avoid safety behaviors.

9. Put it all together and troubleshoot.

STEP ONE: IDENTIFY ACTIVITIES YOU AVOID

You probably have some good ideas of the kinds of activities you tend to avoid because of pain. Make a list of these in your journal. Common examples include driving, lifting, vacuuming, wiping counters, putting away groceries, raking leaves, climbing stairs, carrying a sack of groceries, combing or styling hair, making beds, walking around the block, taking out the trash, bending over to put on shoes, hanging up a heavy coat, putting pet food down, twisting, and dancing. Try to list as many activities as you can, and as above, be specific so there's no doubt what you're referring to.

After you've created your activity list, take a few moments to consider certain sensations that may be emotionally distressing to you other than those that are painful. An example might be a cracking sensation in your neck or a grinding sensation in your back. Many people also find feelings of dizziness, tingling, and numbness worrisome.

STEP TWO: ESTABLISH BASELINES

Before you can establish specific goals for increasing your activity, you need to have a clear idea of your *pain tolerance*—the level of activity that causes significant pain, weakness, or fatigue. Knowing your tolerance level for each activity is important, since it establishes a reference point for beginning your pacing program. You don't want to start too high or too low.

Go through the list of activities you avoid and, in any order, perform each until you feel significant pain, weakness, or fatigue. By *significant*, I mean feeling very uncomfortable but not overwhelmed. When you stop, record the amount of time, frequency, or level of activity you engaged in and write this information in your journal. How you score the activity will depend on the nature of the activity. If you're walking, you could record the amount of time you walked or the distance you traveled. Also record how much your pain interfered with each activity on a scale of 1 to 10, with 10 being the most interference and 1 being the least. Also rate how distressing each of the activities is on a scale of 1 to 10, with 10 being the most distressing or fear producing and 1 being the least.

Monitor your tolerance levels for at least two more days. Don't worry how much your scores fluctuate from day to day and don't attempt to increase how much you do from day to day.

After you've collected your scores, average them across the number of days you monitored. For example, if you walked five minutes on day one, twelve minutes on day two, and seven minutes on day three, the average number of minutes you walked for the three days was eight (5 + 12 + 7 = 24; 24/3 = 8). The average tolerance is called a *baseline score*.

STEP THREE: DEVELOP AN ACTIVITY HIERARCHY

The next step is to rate the activities on your list from least to most difficult. Combine your interference and distress ratings to rank each activity. For example, if you rated bending from the waist as 7 for interference and 8 for distress, the score would be 15. Here's an example of activities arranged hierarchically:

Walking around the block	16
Making the bed	16
Climbing stairs	14
Wiping counters	12
Carrying a sack of groceries	10
Hanging clothes on hangers	8

This hierarchy will come in handy if you have any difficulty in following through on your pacing program. If you start the program and it seems too difficult or you experience too much pain, scale back by eliminating the more challenging activities. After you've experienced some initial success, you can begin to add more difficult items to your program. You may also find it rewarding to go back and rerate each activity in terms of interference and distress after you've been on your pacing program for a while. You'll be pleased to see the scores diminishing with time.

STEP FOUR: SET YOUR INITIAL QUOTAS

Next, you need to determine your initial starting point. You don't want to start at or above your baseline scores since this is the level that's too uncomfortable. The idea is to work toward reasonable goals, not to the point of pain. If you always work to significant pain, you'll look for any excuse to avoid activity. The best approach is to start a little below your baseline. If your distress scores were very high for a particular activity, start even lower to help you gain the confidence you need to stick with your program. You can cut your baseline scores by as much as half if this seems like a reasonable starting point. So if your baseline score for an activity is 8 (eight minutes of walking, for example), you could set your initial quota at 6 or as low as 4.

Don't fret too much about setting your scores so low. Working at or above your baseline tolerance level is very uncomfortable, and if your activity program is too aversive, you'll lose motivation. Although you're unlikely to cause any physical damage by pushing yourself, it will be hard to plug away at the program if you often feel bad. Remember, if pushing yourself to your pain tolerance worked, you'd probably be a lot more active than you are now.

STEP FIVE: SET YOUR TARGET GOAL

Now that you've established your initial quotas, you need to pick a target goal for each activity. This will give you a reasonable end point and set the rate at which you increase your quotas. A rough rule of thumb is to double your baseline levels over a four-week period. So if your baseline score for walking is eight minutes and you want to start at a very low level, you'll increase from four to sixteen minutes of walking over the four-week period. Don't set your target goal too high. You may, more than anything, want to be more active than you are now, but pushing yourself too hard only increases your chances of failing.

STEP SIX: DETERMINE THE RATE OF ACTIVITY INCREASE

Once you've established your baseline scores and target goals, the rest is easy. However, you do need to practice daily, since too much time away from your program will weaken your commitment and make it easier to use excuses and denial to avoid the hard work ahead of you. Practice daily for four weeks, a total of twenty-eight days.

In your journal, sketch out a twenty-eight-day pacing program for each activity, starting at the initial quota and ending up at the target goal. There's no exact formula for you to follow, just bump up your quotas in small increments frequently. The increments need not be evenly spaced. Using the example of increasing walking from four to sixteen minutes daily, your program might look something like this:

Week one (minutes of walking daily): 4, 5, 6, 6, 7, 7, 8

Week two: 8, 9, 9, 9, 10, 10, 10

Week three: 11, 11, 11, 12, 12, 12, 13

Week four: 13, 13, 13, 15, 15, 16, 16

STEP SEVEN: LOG YOUR ACTIVITIES DAILY

The next step in creating your pacing program is to create a log in your journal that you can use to track your progress. List each activity and the quota for that day, and leave a blank space next to each quota to record the level you actually reached that day. You should always try to meet your daily quotas, but there might be days when this isn't possible. Here's an example of a daily log, but you'll probably want to log an entire week per page.

Activities	Mon.
Walking (minutes)	4 _____
Climbing stairs (number of stairs)	6 _____
Doing the dishes (minutes)	2 _____
Lifting from waist to shoulders (pounds)	5 _____
Bending from the waist (degrees)	5 _____
Driving the car (minutes)	10 _____
Using the stationary bike (minutes)	15 _____

STEP EIGHT: IDENTIFY AND AVOID SAFETY BEHAVIORS

The next step is to examine if you engage in any safety behaviors while performing each activity. *Safety behaviors* are subtle forms of avoidance that help you feel safer when you do anything that you believe places you at risk for a worsening of your pain and its consequences. Safety behaviors can also be things you do that you believe help prevent problems from occurring. Here are some examples of safety behaviors reported by my patients:

- Shopping during less crowded times to avoid being knocked over

- Avoiding putting full weight on one leg

- Stepping off a curb or stairs in such a way as to minimize the impact

- Checking your pulse, breathing, level of muscle tension, or other physical signs for reassurance, especially before you commit to engaging in an activity

- Asking friends or loved ones to accompany you when you engage in certain activities or asking them to assist you in tasks you're able to do

- Engaging in activities only when your pain is below average

- Wearing loose clothing to prevent muscle tension

- Limiting activities when you feel too stressed or anxious

- Engaging in activities only at certain times of the day

Identifying your safety behaviors is important since they can undermine your pacing program. By relying upon these subtle forms of avoidance, you are in a sense telling yourself that only under certain conditions can you allow yourself to be active, and that otherwise, you could be putting yourself in jeopardy. Safety behaviors help you feel safer, but you never learn that if you didn't do them nothing terrible would happen.

If, for example, you're only active when you feel relaxed or feel your pain is at its best, you create conditions that reinforce the belief that bad things might have happened if you hadn't engaged in those safety behaviors. You need to teach yourself that you won't lose control of your pain if you don't rely on these strategies.

STEP NINE: PUT IT ALL TOGETHER
AND TROUBLESHOOT

Developing a pacing program is straightforward if you carefully follow the steps outlined above. The most difficult part is troubleshooting problems. A common one is experiencing too much pain when attempting to meet quotas. If this happens, reexamine your program: Did you set your initial quota low enough? Was your target goal too high? Also keep in mind that certain activities will be more distressing than others, and that anxiety about meeting your quotas may be increasing your pain.

If your quotas are realistic and you've set things up properly, try challenging your fearful beliefs about reinjury or exacerbation of pain and then try again. If this doesn't work, lower the rung on the ladder, so to speak, and set your quotas at levels you can definitely achieve. Another possible solution is to start with activities with the lowest interference and distress scores. Once you've increased your confidence, include more difficult activities. Although the order of the hierarchy isn't critical, it might help you initially as you begin your pacing program.

Do whatever is necessary to maximize your success, especially initially. There's no rush. Take your time, don't fight the pain, and try to problem-solve whenever you run into trouble. That said, expect some initial discomfort. Some of this is because you'll start using muscles you haven't used for some time. You'll feel more tight and stiff initially, but this is normal. It's also likely that your pain will increase, since in the past, activity has been associated with pain. This conditioned response is common.

If you can't meet your quota on any particular day, don't feel guilty or despair, just stick to your planned activities the following day. If you can't meet your quota for three consecutive days, reduce the quota, but make sure you understand the reasons you fell short of your quotas (for example, fears of reinjury and pain or unrealistic target goals). Once you've met your initial target goals, decide if you want to continue. You might want to work on only a few of the more important goals. If so, set new targets and persist with your program using the guidelines above.

You may also find that you have trouble eliminating any safety behaviors you're relying on. For example, you may find that fears of falling initially make it too difficult to change your gait, let go of the handrail, put aside your cane, or whatever the case may be. If so, it's okay to wait until your confidence improves, but do set these behaviors aside as you move forward; this will improve your chances for long-term success.

Be aware of any uncomfortable beliefs triggered by increased activity and pain. Challenge these beliefs and learn to lessen their impact by exploring the evidence, as you learned to do in chapter 5. Did your prediction of excruciating pain come true when you were more active? Did you perhaps greatly overestimate the probability that something bad might happen?

▪ Marla's Story

Marla, a thirty-seven-year-old nurse, works for a large hospital in Reno. She was diagnosed with fibromyalgia in her early thirties following a mastectomy and reconstructive surgery. When she was told she had fibromyalgia, she was in the middle of a divorce and had just lost her mother to cancer. Her doctor told her to cut back on her hours and to think about transferring to a less demanding position in the hospital, but Marla resisted because she felt she needed to work and would miss the rewards of clinical nursing.

After several years of trying unsuccessful therapies, including pain pills and antidepressants, Marla was at the end of her rope. Her job was exhausting and exacerbated her pain, leaving her unable to do simple household chores. She called in sick frequently and was running out of excuses. When she came to the pain clinic, she was anxious, depressed, and worried she might lose her job. We used different strategies to help Marla cope with her pain, including developing a pacing program.

As she worked on her pacing program, Marla also challenged her nonproductive thoughts. At first, the idea of attempting to work on any of her quotas was highly distressing, so Marla would wait to do so until she was relatively relaxed and her pain was at or below average. With time, she found she wasn't afraid to work on her easiest quotas in the morning, no matter how she felt. As Marla's confidence increased, she gradually challenged and eliminated most of her safety behaviors. For example, she purposely worked on some of her quotas when she felt most fatigued and stressed. All of these successes defused Marla's anxiety and nonproductive beliefs, allowing her to drop her safety behaviors one by one until they were all eliminated. This helped boost her confidence more than anything. She also noticed that her distress ratings for each activity were considerably lower.

With all of these successes, Marla finally felt comfortable about exposing herself to uncomfortable sensations she had associated with significant physical problems. For example, she worried that the crackling sound when she turned her head back and forth was a sign of serious problems, such as bones grinding against each other. For a long time, she had avoided turning her head and often caught herself turning her entire upper body instead. After reassurances from her physical therapist that this sensation simply indicated tight, tense muscles, Marla started to practice inducing the sensation *purposely. After practicing for only three to five minutes initially, Marla's worrisome thoughts concerning the grinding had disappeared.*

After twenty-eight days, Marla had achieved all of her target goals. Things didn't always go smoothly, and on a couple of occasions she had to go back to the drawing board and revamp her goals. But at the end of the four weeks, she had learned that the negative consequences she expected didn't occur.

Exercise: Review Your Behavior Change Plan

Now would be a good time to return to chapter 2 to review your behavior change goals, as you did at the end of chapter 3. Identify specific activities you'd like to focus on and incorporate them into your behavior change plan. Modify your plan to include overcoming your most troublesome nonproductive beliefs, which you identified in chapter 5.

Increasing your activity level will improve your functioning and overall quality of life. As you begin to do more and realize that past failures can be overcome with persistence and a realistic pacing plan, it's likely that your mood will improve, too. However, conquering negative mood often requires additional work. In chapter 7, you'll learn techniques for enhancing your emotional well-being.

7

Enhancing Your Emotional Well-Being

Chronic pain can take a toll on emotional well-being. It's not difficult to understand why. Chronic pain is associated with numerous losses, a decline in physical fitness, disturbance of sleep, strain on relationships, loss of energy, low activity levels, social isolation and loneliness, and the stress of unremitting pain. Anxiety, depression, and anger are the rule, not the exception, for people in chronic pain. These negative emotions, in turn, exacerbate pain and increase suffering.

Learning to improve your emotional well-being is the focus of this chapter. You might believe this task is too difficult or impossible given all you've experienced. Besides, it's normal to feel upset when pain is constant, and to feel otherwise could be considered abnormal. However, it isn't inevitable that as long as you experience pain there's nothing you can do to feel better emotionally. With some effort, people can learn to feel less depressed, anxious, and angry. In fact, not everyone with chronic pain feels miserable. Although chronic pain increases the risk of emotional turmoil, it isn't an inevitable outcome.

■ Johnny's Story

Johnny was a roofer. Every day he carried heavy bundles of material up tall ladders and laid them out on the rooftops of buildings. For eight to ten hours a day in the hot sun and in the freezing cold of winter he hammered, bent over. He enjoyed the hard work and at the end of the day was physically spent. Johnny made good money and spent it on Jet Skis, snowmobiles, and motorcycles. He said he spent most weekends with his friends, playing hard and "pushing it to the max."

In early spring of 2005, Johnny was walking on a commercial building with a long, sloping roof. Although his boss had warned the crew to use their safety lines, they judged the pitch of the roof safe and decided to forgo them, since they often got in the way when they worked. Early one morning when a thin coat of ice covered parts of the roof, Johnny climbed to the ridge of the roof but then dropped his nail gun. As it slid quickly out of reach, he lunged for it, but his foot suddenly slipped out from under him. He fell on his side and started to slide. He tried to break his momentum by grabbing at anything he could, but he kept picking up speed. He slid over thirty feet before shooting off the edge and slamming into the ground on his buttocks with his legs extended out from him. The fall jackknifed his upper body forward with such force that he hit his knees with his head.

Johnny struggled to his feet to show himself and others he was okay, but excruciating pain in his lower back caused him to buckle over. He drove home but couldn't walk from his truck to his front door and had to yell to his roommate to help him.

After collapsing on the front porch he was taken to the emergency room. An MRI revealed a compression fracture of one of the vertebrae in his lower back, and he was hospitalized for five days.

Johnny's convalescence was difficult. His girlfriend helped him bathe and dress himself for weeks, and since he couldn't go to work, he spent much of his time in bed watching TV. When he tried to increase his activity, his pain flared up, sending him back to bed.

Since Johnny wasn't improving with rest and medication, his family doctor referred him to an orthopedist, who told him there was a 75 percent chance he would respond to a low back surgery. Given the pain and agony he was experiencing, Johnny agreed and the surgery was scheduled. But as he waited for the surgery he started to think that something might go wrong with the operation. He eventually canceled the surgery, telling his doctor he didn't trust that he would have a good outcome.

Johnny admitted later that he decided not to have surgery because he was too anxious. Shortly after his accident, he'd started to have nightmares about falling and was feeling increasingly restless. Images of hitting the ground and the excruciating pain he felt afterward intruded into his waking thoughts, sometimes several times a day, especially when his pain flared up.

Johnny was also getting worried because he wasn't recovering as the doctors had promised he would. He was spending more and more time in bed, since it seemed to be the only way to relieve his pain. When he had to be active, such as shopping for groceries, his pain often flared up, causing him to feel anxious he might have reinjured himself.

*These feelings triggered uncomfortable images and
sometimes symptoms of panic.*

*Five months after his injury, Johnny's pain was
much worse. His girlfriend had broken up with him
and his roommate had moved out, so he was alone
most of the time. His friends had mostly stopped
visiting him because he was irritable and often
snapped at them for things he never used to get upset
over. He was bored and depressed, and his anxiety
symptoms kept worsening. To Johnny, it seemed
everything was falling apart around him. He felt
stuck and had lost what little hope he had that his
situation could ever change for the better.*

How Negative Mood Affects Chronic Pain

Although Johnny's story might seem extreme, it's a familiar one
to many people with chronic pain. Depression afflicts 50 percent
of chronic pain patients (Fishbain et al. 1986), and some have estimated the figure to be much higher (Romano and Turner 1985).
Most experts agree that symptoms of depression occur following
the onset of pain and are more likely to be present in people who
are psychologically susceptible (Sullivan et al. 2001).

As discussed in chapter 1, people with chronic pain seem to
experience more problems with anxiety than the general population (Craig 1994). Fears of reinjury and pain, worries about
future losses (especially of functional abilities and finances),
and a sense of threat of psychological harm from the stress and
strain of chronic pain are common (Rosensteil and Keefe 1983).
Anxiety, when present, contributes to higher levels of distress and
disability associated with chronic pain (Waddell et al. 1993).

Anger is also a frequent problem for many people with chronic pain (Fernandez and Turk 1995). Patients in our clinic often report feeling more irritable and angry after the onset of their pain. Anger, in turn, interferes with activities and increases pain intensity and symptoms of depression (Tearnan and Lewandowski 1992; Kerns, Rosenberg, and Jacob 1994), fueling a vicious cycle. Anger may also significantly interfere with motivation and acceptance of treatment goals in people with chronic pain (Gatchel 2005).

Depression, anxiety, and anger have another debilitating effect: They often make people believe they've changed into someone they don't like—a person who is always angry and discontented, someone indecisive and lacking confidence, a shell of their former self. And in fact, it is difficult to feel or think like your former self when you're depressed, anxious, or angry. However, you haven't lost the things you cherish about yourself—your values and core beliefs. They still reside within you.

Before working on specific techniques to improve your mood, you need to understand the nature of depression, anxiety, and anger. This will help you recognize when you're having problems. Also, bear in mind that negative emotions rarely exist in isolation. When people are angry, they're often depressed and anxious. The suggestions and interventions in this chapter are effective in modifying all three negative emotions.

RECOGNIZING DEPRESSION

Depression, like pain, isn't something you can touch, taste, or smell. Rather, it's defined by a group of symptoms that tend to cluster together when you feel depressed. One useful way of understanding depression is to examine the cognitive (thinking), behavioral, and physiological symptoms that occur with depression.

Cognitive.   When you're depressed, you're likely to report a loss of confidence and feelings of inferiority. You may lose interest in your surroundings and previously pleasurable activities. Motivation declines and many tasks seem to take extra effort. The future often seems bleak, and you may feel hopeless and helpless, so much so that you might entertain thoughts of suicide. You might find it difficult to make decisions and put off doing so, or avoid it altogether. When depressed, you're more likely to be critical of yourself and feel like you've failed or done something wrong. Aaron Beck, a well-known psychiatrist, reported that depressed people adopt a negative and distorted view of themselves, the world around them, and the future (Beck et al. 1979). They often lose the ability to accurately evaluate their experiences, casting everything in a negative hue.

Behavioral.   The primary behavioral change in depression is a reduction in activities, especially pleasant activities. You might stop going out as often and avoid encounters with other people, including family members. Crying can also occur, sometimes at the slightest provocation.

Physiological.   You may experience strong feelings of fatigue, an increase or loss of appetite, disturbance of sleep, or a decline in sexual functioning. You might also complain of more bodily aches and worries about your physical health. In fact, studies have shown that a substantial number of people who report to their doctors with various aches and pains are suffering from depression (Anderson and Anderson 2003).

Not everyone experiences the full spectrum of symptoms known to be associated with depression. People manifest different symptoms, but generally if you notice a significant and prolonged change in your cognitive functioning, you might be depressed. Because most people bothered by persistent pain experience behavioral and physical changes as a consequence of their pain, these categories of symptoms aren't necessarily accurate indicators of depression in people with chronic pain. A decline in activity and changes in sleep, appetite, and energy don't signify depression as reliably as the presence of changes in cognitive functioning (Wesley et al. 1999). More accurate indicators are loss of interest in pleasant activities, especially being around people, feeling worried and discouraged about the future, and self-criticism.

CAUSES OF DEPRESSION IN CHRONIC PAIN

While there are many explanations of how depression develops in chronic pain, most pain experts think that how patients appraise the impact of pain on their lives is important (Turk and Monarch 2002). People who believe they have little control over their pain and its consequences seem to be at higher risk, whereas those who believe they can maintain control and function despite their pain generally don't become depressed.

I often ask my patients if they believe their pain and a good quality of life are incompatible. If they answer yes, I've found there's a strong likelihood of depression. I've also noticed that depression seems to be more common in patients who attribute the problems associated with their pain (for example, financial insecurity, strain on relationships, or loss of a job) to some personal failing. It isn't uncommon for my patients with depression to believe they've failed and are to blame for their problems.

The many losses that can follow the onset of chronic pain also appear to contribute to depression. Most of us are used to dealing with the occasional problem that life throws our way. We confront these difficulties and work our way through them, and eventually most of them resolve or just fade with time. But with chronic pain, you're often challenged by numerous problems that are very stressful and taxing, both physically and emotionally: loss of employment, reduction in activity, social isolation, strain on relationships, uncertainties of medical diagnoses and treatment, and so on. Experiencing so many problems, often in a short span of time, can be overwhelming. In the face of such odds, you might retreat, partly to gather strength, but also because avoidance may seem to be the only way to cope.

Depression is more likely if you believe you aren't up to the challenges you face, or if you attribute negative events to personal shortcomings and begin to believe your life is spinning out of control. Unfortunately, this sort of thinking is common with chronic pain since every effort to overcome pain is met with disappointment and failure. Depression also appears to increase if you believe you've lost important aspects of yourself that you can never retrieve and as a result will never be as happy.

THE IMPORTANCE OF EXPERIENCES THAT COUNTER YOUR BELIEFS

Many people caught in the throes of depression simply give up, often with little hope that their lives will improve. Without experiences to counter the belief that pain and a good quality of life are incompatible, they never learn to reframe the experience of pain. Combating depression requires learning that life can go on despite pain. You can experience more pleasure and a better quality of life, not by recapturing your former self, but by discovering what you can do well and with purpose.

RECOGNIZING ANXIETY

As you'll recall from chapter 1, anxiety occurs in response to threat, real or fantasized. If you believe your pain problem will lead to catastrophic consequences, you'll think and behave in ways consistent with your beliefs. You'll avoid activities you think will aggravate your pain, fearful any increase could push you down the slippery slope of more pain, anxiety, and even panic. For Johnny, aggravation of his pain triggered fearful images and reminders of his traumatic fall. For others, pain is associated with future loss and incapacitation.

When anxiety is attached to pain, pain becomes the center of attention. Fears of dire consequences amplify pain, and the greater a person's expectation of harm, the more severe their perception of pain. To help you understand anxiety's role in your own situation, let's take a closer look at its cognitive, behavioral, physiological, and emotional manifestations.

Cognitive. When we become anxious, our thoughts turn to escape and avoidance. Attention is riveted on reducing the threat. Thoughts are often catastrophic to motivate us to retreat to safety.

Behavioral. Anxiety motivates us to seek safety, usually by avoiding whatever we find threatening. However, anxiety can also provoke you to fight, freeze, or choke.

Physiological. Among the many physiological reactions to anxiety, some of the most common are cold and clammy hands, rapid heartbeat, tense muscles, tingling in the hands and feet, and labored breathing. These physiological responses mobilize the body to fight or flee in the face of the threat.

CAUSES OF ANXIETY IN CHRONIC PAIN

Many things seem threatening to people in chronic pain, and threat is the trigger for anxiety. The vague threats often associated with chronic pain aren't as straightforward as something specific, like a dog snapping at your heels, for example. Because of this, there's uncertainty about whether, when, and how the threat will occur and what can be done if and when it occurs (Lazarus 1994), which can fuel a pervasive apprehensiveness: Will I lose my job? How do I support my family? What if my pain continues to worsen as I age? These threats aren't as easily dismissed and are much more difficult to prepare for than something like an aggressive dog.

RECOGNIZING ANGER

Anger is a common emotional reaction to pain (Turk and Monarch 2002). It's important to talk about since the negative consequences of anger include increased intensity of pain, difficulties in relationships, and higher levels of suffering related to pain (Tearnan and Lewandowski 1992). Chronic anger can also have serious health consequences, including increased risk for heart disease and depression (Hafen et al. 1996). To understand how anger might be affecting you, let's take a look at how it's expressed cognitively, behaviorally, physiologically, and emotionally.

Cognitive. When we're angry, we often feel unfairly slighted and demeaned. Angry people frequently believe their competence and worth is being challenged (Anderson and Anderson 2003). Patients often mention disrespect when talking about what triggers their angry feelings. Anger also appears to be a consequence of being blocked from achieving our goals, even something as simple as fumbling with keys or failing to meet a deadline. I've observed that angry feelings appear stronger when a person invests more importance in a goal and the consequences of failing to achieve that goal.

Behavioral. People express anger in many ways, including hurling insults, hitting objects, using profanity, and fighting. Anger can also be expressed indirectly, such as by being emotionally distant or passively undermining others' efforts.

Physiological. Anger, like anxiety, is a primitive response to threat. It's an important survival mechanism that helps prepare us to defend ourselves. Although we've evolved culturally to the point where anger is usually considered to be an inappropriate response, our bodies still react as our ancestors' did in the face of danger (Hafen et al. 1996). Adrenaline is released, muscles tighten, and the heart beats more rapidly, sending the body a surge of energy and power.

CAUSES OF ANGER IN CHRONIC PAIN

Chronic pain is associated with numerous stressors, including multiple losses and interpersonal conflicts. These stressors often leave people feeling helpless and vulnerable, which can heighten sensitivity about being treated unfairly. You may believe you're powerless to change things and that every attempt to move forward is blocked by unseen forces that you have little or no control over.

Tools for Enhancing Emotional Well-Being

It's misleading and harmful to assume that negative mood is the inevitable consequence of chronic pain and therefore normal. This belief implies that eliminating your pain is the only way you can restore your emotional well-being and reduce your suffering. But in fact, there are many techniques you can use to enhance your emotional well-being in spite of your pain.

In addition to the techniques described below, work on challenging your nonproductive beliefs using the techniques in chapter 5. This will be extremely helpful, as negative unrealistic beliefs can trigger a negative mood. Also consider referring to *The Feeling Good Handbook* by David Burns (1999), an excellent source for understanding and implementing strategies to change nonproductive belief patterns associated with negative mood.

ASSESS YOUR NEGATIVE MOOD

Recognizing your negative moods is important. The self-assessment below will help you determine the degree of depression, anxiety, and anger you're experiencing. It may also help you begin to separate your emotions from your experience of pain. Do this self-assessment weekly so you can track your success with the other techniques described in this chapter. But keep in mind that your mood can fluctuate daily and that this simple self-assessment is not meant to be a diagnostic tool. It simply serves to give you some idea of the intensity of your mood.

Exercise: Self-Assessment

For each statement below, select the one answer that best describes how much you agree or disagree with the statement. For example, if you strongly agree with an item, answer 5, 6, or 7. If you strongly disagree with an item, answer 0, 1, or 2. If you moderately agree or feel neutral about an item, answer 3 or 4.

0   1   2   3   4   5   6   7
Strongly disagree   Strongly agree

DEPRESSION

1.   I feel worthless.   _____

2.   I've lost interest in many things.   _____

3.   I'm sad.   _____

4. I'm discouraged about the future. _____

5. I'm more critical of myself than I used to be. _____

6. I find it difficult to motivate myself to do things. _____

7. I feel tired and run down much of the time. _____

8. I'm dissatisfied with my life. _____

9. I feel inferior. _____

ANXIETY

1. I'm restless. _____

2. It's difficult for me to relax. _____

3. I'm on edge and uptight much of the time. _____

4. My muscles are tense and tight. _____

5. I feel nervous a great deal. _____

6. I often feel stressed. _____

7. My thoughts often seem to race. _____

ANGER

1. I'm often angry. _____

2. I'm frequently irritable. _____

3. I snap at others for the littlest things. _____

4. Everything seems to irritate me. _____

5. I yell at others often. _____

6. I get annoyed with people a lot. _____

7. I often feel resentful toward others. _____

Add up the points for each negative emotion separately. Divide by the total number of questions for that emotion (for example, 7 for anxiety) to reach an average score. A score of 4 or higher suggests that you may be experiencing problems in that area. Write the results in your journal. Complete this questionnaire each week, recording your scores and comparing the results to chart your progress. You can also add all of the items from all three categories to obtain an overall negative mood score. Divide your total score by 23, the total number of items in the questionnaire.

EXERCISE

You've been increasing your activity level using the pacing skills you learned in chapter 6. As you're able to do more and more, your mood will improve, too. Numerous studies have shown that exercise alone can improve mood, especially anxiety and depression. Make sure you choose activities that are fun. For example, if you like to swim, design your activity program to incorporate pool exercises. Remember to start out gradually and work toward reasonable goals.

INCREASE YOUR PLEASANT ACTIVITIES

Studies have also shown that an increase in pleasant activities can improve mood. You may tend to isolate yourself when you feel upset, but this cuts you off from socializing and other pleasant activities, which are essential in maintaining an upbeat mood. Part of the problem is that when we're depressed, angry, or anxious, we often lack motivation and an interest in doing things. The key is to schedule pleasant activities daily and follow through no matter how you feel.

Make a list of all the things you used to like to do for fun or that you're still doing for fun but less frequently. Ask family and friends for ideas or request a copy of the Pleasant Activities Checklist (PACL) on the HealthNetSolutions.com Web site. The PACL is a listing of over three hundred activities most people find positive, rewarding, and useful for enhancing mood. If you develop your own list, try to come up with at least fifty activities. Keep in mind that they should be simple and within your limitations. They should also be activities that you can do daily, or at least weekly. Although going to the beach might be fun, if you live four hundred miles from the coast, this isn't something you can do very often.

Using your list or the PACL, rate each activity on a scale of 1 to 10, with 10 being most pleasant. In your journal, make a new list of only those activities you rated at 8 or above. For one week, use this list to keep a daily log of your pleasant activities by checking off all the activities you engage in each day.

Next, calculate how many pleasant activities you engage in daily on average, then, set a daily goal above your average that you'll try to reach. For example, if your average number of pleasant activities is five, you might want to set an initial daily goal of seven for week one, ten for week two, and so on. Setting daily goals encourages you to plan ahead and schedule your activities. It's best to do so the day before; don't wait until the mood strikes you, because negative mood is the reason you're applying this technique. Your interest in doing things may have waned so much that you'll actually look for excuses to not increase your pleasant activities. Start out slowly, stick to your daily schedule, and get out and have some fun.

If you feel you've done everything right but you're still finding little or no pleasure in the activities you're doing, try examining your thoughts when you're active. You might find that you feel too anxious or self-conscious, or maybe you're choosing activities that are too difficult and physically demanding. Keep going back to the drawing board; and don't give up. It may take a few weeks before you notice an appreciable change in your mood.

TAKE TIME TO RELAX

Negative mood and physiological arousal go hand in hand, especially when you're feeling anxious and angry. Tense muscles, a churning stomach, racing thoughts, and worry are common symptoms reported by people in pain. Learning to relax is a useful skill and one that has been shown to have significant health benefits, including lowering blood pressure and improving sleep.

You may have found that the hardest thing about relaxing is giving yourself permission to sit down quietly and take a few minutes to unwind. You may say to yourself that you're too busy, and you may view relaxation as akin to laziness. Or you might think, "I'm already doing hardly anything as it is. Why would I want to be less active?" Relaxation is not laziness, nor is it doing nothing. It involves active concentration on thoughts, feelings, and bodily sensations and is worthwhile because it promotes a general sense of well-being. It doesn't take a lot of time, and it won't seduce you into wanting to do less and less, as some people fear.

Relaxation will also help you gain more of a sense of personal control, though the reason may sound paradoxical. To relax, you need to learn to feel more comfortable letting go of control. But by letting go of control, you actually put yourself in more control; in a sense you're telling your emotional brain that everything is fine and you aren't in any danger. Otherwise, you wouldn't be letting go! Letting go also is a way of moving toward, not away from, your pain, and this can help counter nonproductive beliefs about negative outcomes. When you truly give up control, you allow yourself to feel whatever comes to you, including your pain. You are in a sense making a very strong statement that the "pain won't hurt me, won't destroy me." The more you learn to relax and feel whatever comes to you, the more you'll be able to tolerate painful sensations instead of believing you have to block them constantly from your awareness.

There are many ways to relax. You're probably already taking time out to passively relax by doing things like listening to music, resting, and taking short walks. However, active relaxation techniques will produce more benefits, including deeper feelings of relaxation and lower levels of muscle tension. Learn a relaxation technique that includes controlled breathing, letting go of muscle tension, and focused concentration. Guided relaxation, slow breathing, and biofeedback, discussed below, are all recommended. But do stay away from progressive muscle relaxation. Although it incorporates all of these aspects and is useful for many people, it requires tensing and releasing various muscle groups, which can trigger more pain in people with chronic pain problems.

Relaxation therapy is best if practiced daily. During your relaxation practice, turn off your phone and ask others not to disturb you. Set aside the countless things that must be done and give yourself permission to enjoy the benefits of letting go and relaxing.

GUIDED RELAXATION

Guided relaxation techniques that use suggestions for warmth and letting go of muscle tension are ideal. I often use the following script with my patients. Make a tape of it using your own voice, or ask a family member or friend to make a recording of it. Read the words slowly and pause often. You can also order a prerecorded tape on the HealthNetSolutions.com Web site.

> *Let yourself get as comfortable as you can. Now scan your body with your mind's eye and pay attention to any areas of tightness or tension. Let yourself focus on those areas. Don't try to rid yourself of any tension right now. Just let those feelings be as they are; don't try to push them away.*
>
> *Now focus your attention on the muscles of your scalp. Imagine those muscles becoming relaxed, quiet, and calm. Just put your mind's eye to the top of your head and feel those muscles loosening up a bit. Now bring your attention to the muscles of your forehead ... Let the lines of tension in the muscles of your forehead smooth themselves out ... Let the relaxation spread to the muscles of your temples, your eyes, even the backs of your eyes ... Now let the relaxation seep into the muscles of your jaw, letting your teeth part slightly so the muscles of your jaw begin to relax. Let go of the tension in the muscles around your cheeks, your lips, your tongue, even your throat ... Just let all the muscles of your face let go and relax ... Now pay attention to the muscles in the back of your head. Feel the muscles loosening slowly. Feel yourself becoming more calm and quiet ... Let the muscles of your neck relax as well. If you're lying down, your head is completely supported, so there's no reason to tense or to move*

the muscles of your neck. Just let yourself go as much as you can. Don't force the relaxation—just let it come to you. Don't chase any particular feeling. Just relax as much as you can, and no more ... Now pay attention to your shoulder muscles. Feel the tightness begin to ease itself. Feel the tension begin to give way ... Deeper and deeper—more deeply relax. Ease the tension away, letting yourself feel calm and quiet and at ease ... let go of the tension in the muscles of your upper arms, your forearms, hands, and fingers, slowly letting go, more and more ... deeply relaxed, calm, and quiet. Feel the tension begin to ease itself out of your muscles. Let yourself begin to feel a sense of heaviness and warmth flowing into your muscles—heavy, warm, and relaxed ... Let the relaxation spread into the muscles of your fingers. Just let go as much as you can, no more ... Now let your attention focus on the muscles of your chest and stomach. Let your breathing be the only thing that lifts and moves the muscles of your chest and stomach ... slowly in a circular pattern ... rhythmically breathing in and out. Each time you breathe out, feel a sense of relaxation flow into the muscles of your chest and stomach. Feel yourself let go with each breath—quiet and calm—more and more relaxed ... Now turn your attention to the muscles of your upper back. Feel the tension begin to ease itself out of the muscles of your back. Let the relaxation spread into the muscles of your mid back, running slowly down to your lower back and buttocks. Just let go and completely relax, giving up as much tension as you can and no more ... Let the tension begin to drift away from the muscles in your thighs and now the muscles of your calves, your ankles, and down to your feet, even the bottoms of your feet. Let all the muscles of your legs begin to relax. Let yourself feel quiet, calm, and at ease.

Say to yourself, "The muscles in my legs are beginning to feel heavy, warm, and relaxed. The muscles in my lower back and buttocks are beginning to relax. My muscles are feeling more quiet and calm. The muscles of my mid back and upper back are letting go of tension. The muscles of my stomach and chest are beginning to let go. My breathing is smooth and even, like a circle. Every time I breathe out, I feel myself relax more and more. The muscles in my arms are beginning to feel heavy, warm, and relaxed. Quiet and calm ... releasing tension ... letting go. The muscles in my shoulders are letting go of tension, deeper and deeper ... more deeply relaxed. The tension is slowly fading away. The muscles in my neck are letting go of tension. They're beginning to feel heavy—so heavy, warm, and relaxed. The muscles in the back of my head and scalp are relaxing, feeling smooth, still, and at ease. The muscles in my face are letting go of tension ... quiet and calm. My mind is beginning to feel at ease—deeply relaxed, slowly letting go ... becoming more and more quiet and calm."

Just let go—let go completely. Completely relax. Now focus your attention on the number 20. I'm going to count backwards from 20 to 1, and as I count backwards, I want you to feel more and more relaxed, more quiet and calm. By the time I reach 0, you will have let go of even more tension, as much as you can. Don't force the tension away, just let go as much as you are able to ... 20 ... deeper and deeper, more deeply relaxed ... 19 ... just let go, more and more ... 18 ... quiet and calm ... more deeply relaxed ... 17 ... just let go ... 16 ... 15 ... 14 ... deeper and

*deeper ... 13 ... quiet and calm and at ease ... 12 ...
just feel yourself begin to give up tension, not forcing
it, just feeling yourself drift, quiet and calm, letting
your mind go wherever it wants to go but still able to
hear my voice ... 11 ... 10 ... 9 ... deeper and deeper,
more deeply relaxed ... just let yourself go ... 8 ... 7 ...
deeper and deeper, more deeply relaxed ... 6 ... 5 ...
quieter and calmer ... 4 ... just let go, more and more
... 3 ... 2 ... feel yourself ease ever more deeply into
relaxation, quiet and calm, deeper and deeper, more
deeply relaxed ... 1 and 0, letting go completely.
Completely relaxed, quiet, calm, and at ease. Just
let yourself be at peace. Let yourself relax. Feel the
enjoyment of being quiet, of being calm. Let yourself
ease into relaxation, deeper and deeper, more deeply
relax. Just let go.*

SLOW BREATHING

A shorter way of relaxing is to simply slow your breathing down and breathe deeply. Sit in a comfortable position and
breathe in slowly. Use diaphragmatic breathing, in which your
abdomen rises with each inhalation, not your chest. Breathe in
through your nose for three to four seconds, hold for about two
seconds, then slowly breathe out through your mouth as if you
were cooling hot soup on a spoon. If your breathing feels strained,
pick up the pace a bit. The keys are to breathe slowly and evenly,
to concentrate your attention on your breath, and to feel yourself
becoming calmer and more at ease each time you exhale.

BIOFEEDBACK

Biofeedback uses instrumentation to monitor different
physical processes, such as heart rate, brain wave activity, muscle

tension, and skin temperature, using sensors that detect electrical signals produced by the body. These signals are transmitted to a biofeedback machine and transformed into an auditory or visual form. With practice, people can learn to control their physiology using this visual or auditory information. Biofeedback is used to treat various painful conditions, including headaches. It's also used to promote a general state of relaxation by teaching patients to control muscle tension and reduce their fight-or-flight response.

ENGAGE IN MASTERY EXPERIENCES

Chronic pain often leaves people feeling helpless. Sometimes nothing seems to fall into place and everything seems doomed to fail. You may have a sense of disconnection from your environment and feel powerless to alter your world to make it right again.

The best way to combat these beliefs is not by giving in and not adopting what I call the "chronic pain holding pattern": circling, waiting to land, forever removed from everyday life. Instead, you need to engage in experiences that teach you what you say and do still makes a difference. Keep in mind that when a negative mood takes hold, distorted thinking rules the day and you're more likely to believe the negative side of things. So you stay stuck, accepting things as they are and believing that nothing will change.

Mastery experiences can shake your thinking out of its well-worn groove and affirm that what you do still counts. Mastery experiences differ from person to person. They're what makes you feel good about yourself and your importance. The following exercise will help you brainstorm and come up with experiences that can challenge your sense of helplessness.

Exercise: Choosing Mastery Experiences

Use the list of mastery experiences below as a starting point for generating a list more pertinent to you. Pick those activities you think will help counter your beliefs of helplessness and add anything else that suggests itself to you.

- Meeting your daily pacing goals

- Having a lively or open and frank talk with family or friends

- Playing chess, checkers, or other games

- Writing a letter to an old friend

- Helping someone or volunteering in your community

- Building something

- Making a special meal

- Painting a picture, doing crafts, playing music, and other creative endeavors

- Driving skillfully

- Suggesting to your doctor or physical therapist something you might try, such as a new exercise

- Cleaning or redecorating a room

- Paying bills

- Working in your garden

MANAGE YOUR FATIGUE

Nearly everyone with chronic pain battles fatigue daily. A number of factors can affect your energy level, including stress, boredom, lack of sleep, poor nutrition, physical deconditioning, and many of the medications that are prescribed for chronic pain. But a negative mood can also be a major factor. When you're anxious, depressed, or angry, you lose motivation and your interest in doing things. This may be due, in part, to a belief that nothing matters and there's no use in trying, since nothing good will come of it.

Simply knowing that negative mood can impact energy levels can help you counteract its effects. Examine what you used to enjoy doing and why, and trust this information rather than succumbing to the belief that nothing matters and why bother.

To increase your energy levels, start by talking with your doctor about your medications to determine whether anything you're taking might be causing excessive fatigue or disrupting your sleep. Speak with your doctor about your nutrition as well. Eating three meals a day and the right kinds of healthy snacks can energize your body.

Next, focus on your activity program and improve your physical conditioning. As you do more and increase your strength and endurance, you'll notice your energy level slowly returning. To combat boredom, which can lead to low energy levels, try to incorporate interesting and stimulating activities in your day-to-day routine. Boredom often plagues people with chronic pain, especially those who have stopped doing many things.

And finally, though it may seem obvious, don't overlook the possibility that you're not getting enough sleep. A good night's sleep is essential to feeling energized, and also essential to managing your pain. Chapter 8 is devoted to this important topic.

TO MEDICATE OR NOT

Numerous medications are prescribed for depression and anxiety. Despite their enormous popularity, they aren't effective for all people and most have the potential for bothersome side effects. You can definitely improve your mood without the use of antidepressants or other medications, including tranquilizers. Antidepressants, as an example, aren't essential treatments for mood enhancement but may prove useful for some. Even so, most pain experts agree that when antidepressants are used for treating depression, they should be combined with other therapies, including some of the techniques discussed in this chapter.

SEEK PROFESSIONAL HELP

Negative mood can have an enormous impact on pain, activity levels, sleep, general health, relationships, and work. Fortunately, there's much you can do on your own to effect a change in your mood and turn your life around. This chapter, and books such as *The Feeling Good Handbook* by David Burns (1999), can help tremendously, but sometimes it may be necessary to seek the counsel of a psychologist or other mental health professional, especially if you feel hopeless to the extent that you've contemplated suicide or you find that your mood is severely disrupting many aspects of your life. You should also consider consulting a professional if you've given the strategies in this book a good effort but are still experiencing moderate to severe levels of mood disturbance.

A good place to start is to ask your family doctor or a trusted friend for a reference. The Internet is also useful, especially for contacting mental health professionals who specialize in the treatment of chronic pain. Or contact the American Pain Society or the American Academy of Pain Management, two professional organizations that can help you locate mental health pain specialists in your area.

A wide variety of techniques can help you overcome depression, anxiety, and anger, and you have every reason to feel optimistic about eventually achieving a change in your mood. As you practice the techniques in this chapter, try to identify which work best for you. You may find that you prefer certain ones, or that some of them are preferable in specific situations. Because mood and energy levels are significantly impacted by sleep problems, which are so prevalent in chronic pain, chapter 8 is devoted to strategies to help you get to sleep and stay asleep.

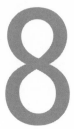

Improving Your Sleep

It may have been a long time since you slept well. Pain, stress, and adjusting to the problems caused by chronic pain can take their toll on a good night's sleep. In our clinic, nearly 85 percent of pain patients have problems with insomnia. Their sleep disturbance is frequently complicated by medical problems other than pain, such as obesity and sleep apnea, and by psychological problems that are often due to pain, such as depression, anger, and anxiety. In many cases, medications used to treat pain problems—including narcotics, tranquilizers, and muscle relaxers—are partially and sometimes significantly responsible for aggravating sleep disturbance.

As you read this chapter, you may be surprised to learn that some of the things you're doing in an effort to improve your sleep may be backfiring and causing you further problems. This chapter will help you identify poor sleep habits and replace them with simple, effective techniques that will help.

■ Karl's Story

Karl's back pain started after shoveling snow two years ago. He complained of a dull ache and sharp pains in his lower back and buttocks. Tylenol and rest gave him some relief, but only for a few hours. After three weeks in near-constant pain, he went to see his family doctor, who prescribed Vicodin (hydrocodone with acetaminophen) and an anti-inflammatory medication. This helped ease his pain, but not consistently.

When he returned for a follow-up visit, Karl told his doctor he was having trouble sleeping. He had always been a sound sleeper, but since he injured his back, he tossed and turned and would wake up several times each night. Sometimes he would lie awake for hours before falling into a fitful sleep.

He tried using over-the-counter sleeping medications, but these only made him feel groggy and hungover the next morning, so his doctor prescribed Ambien (zolpidem), a short-acting tranquilizer for sleep. At first the Ambien worked wonders. Karl was finally able to fall asleep within minutes and usually stayed asleep for several hours. But after a few weeks he started waking up early in the morning and couldn't get back to sleep.

Karl said he often stared at his bedside clock, trying to force himself to sleep. If midnight passed he worried the next day would be rough, and if he was still awake by 2:00 a.m., he was convinced the next day would be shot. He couldn't get the thought out of his head that if he didn't get a good night's sleep, his job performance would suffer from his lack of concentration and fatigue.

When Karl came to our clinic, he was averaging three hours of uninterrupted sleep per night. It took him more than two hours to fall asleep, and he woke up five to six times during the night. He described his sleep quality as "lousy" and complained of daytime fatigue, problems concentrating, and grogginess from the residual effects of Ambien, and he was depressed because he couldn't get a solid night's sleep.

Sleeping Pills

Good sleep is possible if you have chronic pain, but achieving a restful night's sleep involves much more than taking a pill. In fact, taking sleeping pills may be part of why you don't sleep well.

Most of the prescription sleeping pills on the market are benzodiazepines, a class of drugs more commonly known as tranquilizers. When you first start to use them, they'll help you get to sleep and stay asleep, but they have a serious downside: They decrease deep sleep and frequently cause daytime drowsiness, concentration problems, and negative mood. They can also cause both physiological and psychological dependency. Newer, shorter-acting benzodiazepines have fewer side effects, but many people who take them often awaken in the middle of the night and can't get back to sleep. Dependency is a problem with these newer drugs, too. Imidazopyridines are another, even newer sleeping aid, with yet fewer side effects and problems with dependency. But like the newer benzodiazepines, they're not as effective at helping people stay asleep throughout the night—a problem that particularly afflicts people in chronic pain.

Older classes of antidepressants—tricyclics and tetracyclics— are also commonly used to treat insomnia, especially in people with chronic pain. Although they weren't developed to treat sleep disturbances, they cause significant sedation in most people.

When prescribed as hypnotics or sleep aids, they're given at doses well below the levels considered effective for treating depression. These drugs can shorten the time it takes to fall asleep and help people stay asleep. They can also provide mild pain relief, especially with nerve injuries. However, many people can't tolerate the side effects these drugs can cause, even at very low doses, such as daytime sedation, dry mouth, blurred vision, problems urinating, constipation, and weight gain. In addition, they can lose their effectiveness within a relatively short period and may cause psychological dependence. On the upside, they don't produce withdrawal effects when stopped abruptly, and they don't interfere with deep sleep (Jacobs 1998).

In the past decade, over-the-counter sleeping aids have become increasingly popular. Most contain an antihistamine as the active ingredient. There's no evidence, however, that these drugs are any more effective than placebos for treating chronic insomnia, and they often have side effects similar to the antidepressants. They can also heighten anxiety and disrupt REM sleep (Dement 1999). Herbal and other sleep aids, such as melatonin, valerian root, kava, and L-tryptophan, are also available over the counter, but there's no strong evidence that they produce lasting relief from chronic insomnia.

Many of the medications used to control pain, including narcotics, anticonvulsants, and muscle relaxers, can cause sedation, so patients and physicians often view them as sleep aids. Unfortunately, these drugs often disrupt sleep, cause uncomfortable side effects, and ultimately exacerbate insomnia.

The problem with sleeping pills is that they don't address the underlying problems so often associated with insomnia, including anxiety about not sleeping, poor sleep habits, and conditioning (Hauri and Linde 1996; Jacobs 1998). However, when used judiciously for short periods, and in combination with techniques discussed below, they can be part of an effective sleep management program for people with chronic pain.

TECHNIQUES FOR IMPROVING SLEEP

Pain and physical discomfort often cause poor sleep, which, unfortunately, is often made worse by the very things people do to restore a good night's sleep, including using sleeping pills and some widely practiced treatments for pain. To improve your sleep, you need to relearn how to sleep well. This means understanding and changing the things that have contributed to poor sleep and learning effective techniques for improving sleep. Let's take a look at some of the techniques that have proven helpful for people with chronic pain.

ASSESS YOUR SLEEP

Before you start working with the techniques in this chapter, copy the daily sleep log below into your journal so you can track important aspects of your sleep on a daily basis. Each morning, take a couple of minutes to record your answers so you can see if your efforts are making a difference in your sleep from week to week.

Exercise: Daily Sleep Log

Date: _____

1. Approximately how much total time did you spend in bed last night, sleeping or just lying in bed? ____

2. Approximately how many total hours did you sleep? ____

3. Approximately how long did it take for you to fall asleep? ____

4. How many times did you
   awaken during the night?   _____

5. What was the longest time it
   took for you to fall back asleep? _____

6. What time did you wake up in
   the morning?   _____

7. Did you nap yesterday? Yes _____
   No _____ If yes, for how long
   and at what time of day?

   _____

8. What was the overall quality of
   your sleep last night from 0 to 7,
   with 0 being very poor and 7
   being very good?   _____

9. List any medications, including
   any over-the-counter drugs, you
   used for sleep: _____

10. Rate your overall level of tension
    or anxiety during the night from
    0 to 7, with 0 being no tension or
    anxiety, and 7 being very high
    tension or anxiety: _____

   Your daily sleep log will also help you understand any fluctuations in your sleep pattern. This
will prove useful when you begin to examine
factors that could be influencing your sleep (for
example, stress and anxiety).

MODIFY YOUR SLEEP ENVIRONMENT

Take a few minutes to think about your bedroom and what you could do to improve your sleep environment. This can include simple things like pulling the shades down at night or getting darker curtains to block the early morning light. Adjust the temperature of your bedroom if you're too cold or warm. If neighborhood noise is keeping you awake, turn on a fan or buy a white noise generator to mask the sound. Get a comfortable pillow and use more than one if this helps you position your body more comfortably. Think about adjusting your mattress or buying a new one if you believe this will help. Be creative and brainstorm what you can do to modify your sleep environment to facilitate your sleep.

TAKE ADVANTAGE OF GOOD CONDITIONING

Good sleep is a natural physiological process. However, it's also true that people who sleep well are conditioned to good sleep. A bedtime routine, the bed, the time of day, and even thoughts help promote sound sleep. If, for example, your bed is strongly associated with tiredness and relaxation, you're more likely to fall asleep and sleep soundly. If, however, you watch TV in bed or toss and turn while trying to force yourself to sleep, your bed can become conditioned to wakefulness, disrupting the sleep process. This is why many insomniacs can be exhausted and sleepy but feel wide awake as soon as they lie down.

Your bed should be associated with sleepiness, not wakefulness. Don't go to bed until you're tired. When you go to bed, don't watch TV, listen to the radio, or read in bed. If you do, limit this time to fifteen minutes or less. You want your bed to be a trigger for sleep, not wakefulness.

It's also important that you allow no more than thirty minutes to fall asleep. This should be your subjective judgment of how much time has elapsed. Don't watch the clock; in fact, turn your clock around. You don't need to know the time once the lights are off, and don't check the clock when you awaken at night. This will only heighten your anxiety about not sleeping.

If you can't fall asleep within thirty minutes, get out of bed and do something monotonous until you feel sleepy and then return to bed. If, once again, you can't fall asleep within thirty minutes, repeat the process. Avoid activities that might be stimulating, such as checking your e-mail, catching up on work, composing a letter, or exercising. During your time out of bed, don't fall asleep in your recliner or on the couch, especially if this is habitual for you. Wait until you're sleepy, then return to your bed.

Just as your bed can be a cue for sleep, the activities you engage in before bedtime can also send strong cues to your body and brain that sleep is around the corner. Here are a few suggestions you might consider incorporating into a regular bedtime routine:

- Take a warm bath an hour or two before bedtime.

- Practice your relaxation exercises before you go to bed.

- Read, but not in bed.

- Drink a cup of calming noncaffeinated herbal tea.

CHALLENGE YOUR ANXIOUS THOUGHTS ABOUT NOT SLEEPING

Once poor sleep has become a problem, many people can't fall asleep because they worry about not sleeping. As soon as you hit the pillow, your mind may shift into overdrive with worrisome thoughts about whether it will be a good night. You might find yourself monitoring every nuance of tension or pain and whether you're moving closer to or farther from sleep.

Being able to fall asleep in a relatively short span of time requires a relaxed brain, especially when you're in constant pain. You have to put aside your worries about not sleeping. Sometimes nothing seems to matter more than getting a good night's sleep, but it's important to take the pressure off yourself. I bet you can remember times when you had an awful night's sleep but still had a pretty good day afterward. People can go a long time without a good night's sleep without serious emotional or physical ill effects. Getting a good night's sleep is obviously the goal and it will make you feel better, but don't convince yourself that disastrous consequences will occur, including an aggravation of your pain, if you don't sleep well, even for several days or weeks.

Exercise: Your Thoughts About Sleep

Take a look at the following list of thoughts common to people with chronic pain who have difficulty sleeping. Examine the evidence, as you did in chapter 5, and challenge each one until you can confidently say to yourself, "There's no proof, data, or fact to support that thought."

- If I don't get to sleep on time, the next day will be shot.

- If I don't get a good night's sleep, my pain will flare up.

- If I don't get a good night's sleep, I'll be depressed.

- If I don't sleep well, my health will suffer terribly.

One thing I often recommend to my patients with sleep problems is to try to stay awake when they turn the lights out at night. Reverse psychology? Sure it is. But give it a try. Put your heart and soul into staying awake. If you're successful, it will help convince you that the consequences of staying awake aren't terrible or catastrophic. It might even help you fall asleep more quickly!

LEARN TO MANAGE YOUR STRESS

In chapter 7 you learned some relaxation skills. These techniques can also help you sleep more soundly. Relaxation calms anxious thoughts and tense, tight muscles. Use the tape you made or purchased and play it before you go to bed to help you relax.

RESTRICT YOUR TIME IN BED

Maximizing wakefulness during the day is an important part of getting a good night's sleep (Jacobs 1998). To accomplish this, reduce the amount of time you spend in bed to the amount of time you actually sleep. (But don't go below five and a half hours, which Jacobs says is necessary to ensure *core sleep*, the amount of deep sleep necessary for maximum daytime performance.) For example, if your daily sleep log shows you're averaging six hours of sleep a night but spend nine hours in bed, reduce the time you're in bed to six hours. To determine the time you should go to bed, set a firm wake-up time and subtract your average sleep time plus one hour. So if you want to wake up at six and you're sleeping six hours on the average, you'd go to bed at eleven. Don't go to bed until your predetermined time, no matter how tired you feel. Also, make sure you wake up at the time you've set every day, even on weekends. If you nap, take only short naps (for example, thirty minutes). Some sleep experts recommend napping no later than late afternoon so as not to affect your nighttime sleep.

Restricting time in bed as a treatment for insomnia was originally developed by Art Spielman, a psychologist at City College of New York. The goal of this approach is to improve your sleep efficiency to at least 85 percent. *Sleep efficiency* is calculated by dividing your average sleep time by the total time you spend in bed. Once you've improved to at least 85 percent for two weeks, increase your time in bed by fifteen minutes each week. Using the example above, you would start to go to bed at 10:45 after achieving 85 percent efficiency for two weeks, and so on.

CHANGE YOUR CIRCADIAN RHYTHM

Many of the body's functions are regulated on a twenty-four-hour internal clock called the *circadian rhythm*, including sleep and wake times. If you're sleeping at times you don't want to sleep, your circadian rhythm may be out of sync. For example, if you sleep well from 1 a.m. to 9 a.m. but can't sleep when you go to bed at 10 p.m., your circadian rhythm may be disordered, at least in relation to your ideal sleep schedule. Regulating your circadian rhythm will improve your chances of sleeping.

If you believe your circadian rhythm is disordered because you sleep well at times you don't want to sleep, you may be experiencing delayed or advanced sleep phase syndrome. Restricting your time in bed and setting a firm wake-up time will help, but you may be fighting an uphill battle if your internal clock is out of sync with your desired sleep time. *Delayed sleep phase syndrome* occurs when you typically fall asleep late (for instance, 3 a.m.) and sleep late. *Advanced sleep phase syndrome* involves going to sleep much earlier than desired (for instance, 6 p.m.) and waking up much earlier.

Some sleep experts recommend using *phototherapy*, or light therapy, to correct circadian rhythm disorder (Jacobs 1998; Hauri and Linde 1996). If you have delayed sleep phase syndrome, expose yourself to sunlight or indoor light for about an hour as soon as you wake up in the morning. If you use indoor light, it should put out between 5,000 to 10,000 lux. (So-called bright light boxes can be purchased from various companies.) This exposure to light decreases levels of melatonin, a hormone found in the brain. This causes your body temperature to rise earlier than normal, shifting your internal clock so that you become sleepy earlier. If you think you have advanced sleep phase syndrome, expose yourself to bright light or sunlight right after your evening meal. This will result in a decrease in melatonin and delay the onset of sleep.

Phototherapy can dramatically improve a fast or slow internal clock, but you must consistently expose yourself to light at the appropriate time daily. Once your sleep improves, usually after two to three weeks, you can reduce the amount of light exposure, but you may find that some phototherapy is still needed to keep your internal clock regulated.

INCREASE YOUR PHYSICAL ACTIVITY

Sleep improves with physical activity. One reason people with chronic pain experience sleep problems is a sharp reduction in activity. Activity also helps dissipate the effects of stress, which are so common to the chronic pain experience. Stress hormones produced by the brain to sustain the fight-or-flight response are depleted with physical activity, resulting in a more relaxed mental and physical state.

Although increasing your activity level will help you sleep, it could exacerbate your pain. Follow the recommendations for pacing in chapter 6, and try to pick activities that energize your whole body and get your heart pumping. Walking and swimming are good exercises for most people with pain. Ask your doctor or physical therapist for suggestions. Remember to start gradually and set realistic goals.

USE SLEEPING MEDICATIONS WISELY

If you decide to use a sleeping medication, make sure your choice is one of the new imidazopyridines or, preferably, a tricyclic antidepressant. Use the medication only as an initial boost to help you start your sleeping program and then gradually wean yourself from the medication after you've met your sleeping goals. Try not to rely upon medications for more than a few weeks, and always combine the other techniques in this chapter with any use of medication, since the pills by themselves are unlikely to work in the long term. Learning to sleep without medication will boost your confidence and strengthen your ability to sleep.

AVOID STIMULANTS

Last, but certainly not least, avoid stimulants, especially caffeine, which is present in tea, sodas, and chocolate, as well as coffee. If you consume caffeinated drinks, try not to have them after midday. Certain activities and experiences can also be highly stimulating and interfere with your sleep, such as vigorous exercise, video games, or certain types of movies, television shows, and music. Try to avoid these types of stimulating activities in the hours leading up to bedtime, too.

Keep in mind it will take time to restore your sleep. Don't expect overnight success and be prepared to go back to the drawing board more than once to improve your sleep program. With a little effort and a commitment to change, you will succeed. Also consider consulting one or more of the many excellent books for treating insomnia, such as *Say Good Night to Insomnia* by Gregg Jacobs (1998).

Exercise: Review Your Behavior Change Plan

Just as you did at the end of chapters 3 and 6, take a few minutes to review the behavior change goals you established in chapter 2. Are you meeting your goals? What adjustments and additions do you need to make? Perhaps you'd like to add some goals related to improving your sleep habits. If you're running into problems, try to troubleshoot what you can do to improve things. Remember to pace yourself, keep your expectations realistic, and motivate yourself by maximizing the gains and minimizing costs.

Improving sleep requires that you pay attention to both psychological and biological aspects of sleep. Hopefully all of the techniques you've learned up to this point in the book have brought you significant relief and an improved quality of life. However, it may be that you still need pain medications or other forms of medical intervention, or perhaps your doctor still encourages these methods of treatment. Chapter 9 will give you background information on the various biomedical treatments for managing both acute and chronic pain to help you make informed decisions about this important but complex issue.

9

Considering Biomedical Treatments

B iomedical treatments are the first line of defense in the treatment of acute pain. They're used to promote healing and alleviate discomfort. They're curative and designed to alter physical pain-generating mechanisms, such as a compressed nerve or strained muscle. In chronic pain, however, biomedical approaches have proven to be singularly ineffective in addressing the range of problems most people experience. Despite this, when combined with cognitive and behavioral therapies, biomedical treatments can be highly useful in the management of chronic pain.

The overriding goal of biomedical therapies for chronic pain is to encourage movement and relaxation in tight, deconditioned muscles and to provide symptomatic relief of pain when possible through physical, chemical, electrical, and surgical treatments. This chapter focuses on the most commonly used biomedical approaches for treating chronic pain. As discussed throughout this book, knowledge is power, and in the case of medical treatments, being better informed puts you in charge of your care and enables you to more effectively communicate with your doctors so that you can ask the right questions and expect more—and sometimes less.

Physical Therapies

The physical therapies applied in the treatment of chronic pain are designed primarily to affect the musculoskeletal system and include most types of physical therapy, chiropractic manipulation, exercise, and massage. Since chronic pain is generally associated with limited range of motion and diminished strength, the thrust of physical therapies is to increase flexibility, strength, and, with time, endurance. Let's take a look at some of the more popular methods used in the physical treatment of chronic pain.

STRETCHING

Muscle atrophy from disuse can impact your entire musculoskeletal system. As a result, stretching your arms and legs is important even if your pain is limited to your lower back, for example. Every physical therapist teaches general stretching.

Far fewer therapists teach trigger point stretches, even though trigger points are present in a majority of patients with chronic pain (Travell and Simons 1992). These exquisitely tender points in the muscle tend to occur in specific locations in any given muscle. Trigger points are associated with referred pain that's distant from the site of the trigger point itself. Referred pain is a common phenomenon associated with muscle pain. A heart attack causing pain to the left arm or back is a good example of referred pain.

Although trigger points are common in chronic pain, their physical cause remains unknown, although theories abound. As painful and debilitating as trigger points can be, they aren't linked to any disease or serious physical malady. Surprisingly, a muscle with trigger points is generally healthy.

If you think you have trigger points, ask your doctor or physical therapist to conduct a trigger point exam. If they don't know how, ask for a referral to a physical therapist or physician familiar with trigger point therapies.

Physical therapists and physicians differ considerably when recommending how frequently muscles with trigger points should be stretched. Some recommend stretching five times a day, whereas others suggest hourly stretching, at least initially. They also differ regarding the duration of stretching, with some recommending a ten-second stretch and others twenty seconds or longer. However, all agree stretching should be done slowly, gently, and never to the point of pain.

In our clinic, patients are given handouts of the muscles where trigger points have been identified. They're taught to stretch their muscles with trigger points at least five times a day for fifteen to twenty seconds each, using breathing and good body posture while completing the stretch. They're also taught to stretch to the point of tension, never pain. A physician measures the activity of trigger points weekly, and if needed, trigger point injections are applied.

TRIGGER POINT INJECTIONS

Trigger point injections involve injecting a local anesthetic directly into the trigger point. Although the injections are painful, they can provide temporary relief from pain, allowing the muscle to be more easily stretched, the most important ingredient in treating trigger points. Not everyone responds well to trigger point injections. Some people show little or no reaction, while others complain that the injections are too painful and aggravate their pain. Physicians sometimes combine the local anesthetic with steroids, but there's no strong evidence that trigger points are an inflammatory condition and therefore steroids are generally not recommended.

Immediately after giving trigger point injections, the practitioner stretches the target muscles to their full passive range of motion. Trigger point injections by themselves are unlikely to benefit you if not combined with stretching. Sometimes physicians also recommend deep massage after trigger point injections.

ACUPUNCTURE

Some physicians use acupuncture to treat trigger points. Tiny needles are inserted directly into the trigger points, and sometimes electrical stimulation is applied to the tip of the needle after it's inserted. However, there's no evidence that electricity adds to the effectiveness of acupuncture. Traditional acupuncture is also sometimes used for chronic pain. In this case, acupuncture needles are inserted into the muscles at acupoints, key locations that occur on meridians of energy postulated to exist by practitioners of this ancient Chinese healing technique. Interestingly, these overlap considerably with known locations of trigger points.

As with trigger point injections, acupuncture has mixed success in treating chronic pain. Both are termed *counterirritant therapies* since they apply a painful stimulus to a trigger point. Some physicians also practice dry needling, a technique in which a syringe needle containing only saline solution is inserted into a trigger point, producing effects very similar to acupuncture needling.

ACUPRESSURE

In acupressure, another counterirritant therapy, sustained pressure is applied, usually with the fingers, to acupoints or trigger points for up to a minute or longer. Although it's difficult, you can apply it to yourself if your trigger points are conveniently located, especially in your arms and legs. Some people use a tennis ball against a wall or the floor, or you can lean against the threshold of a door to achieve the same effect as a therapist's firm finger pressure.

As with most of the physical therapies for chronic pain, acupressure may or may not help. The approach most practitioners take is to try a particular technique to see if it's successful, especially in whether it helps increase movement and relaxation of the muscle and deactivation of trigger points.

MASSAGE

Most people with chronic pain respond favorably to massage, which can help promote relaxation of tense muscles. However, some massage techniques can aggravate chronic pain, especially when applied to muscles with painful trigger points or if you have difficulty tolerating any touch or pressure. Although massage can produce relief, it's usually temporary and it requires a passive dependence on others. It can also be expensive. However, treating yourself to an occasional massage can be rewarding and will help remind you of the benefits of muscle relaxation.

CHIROPRACTIC MANIPULATION

Chiropractic manipulation can provide temporary relief of chronic pain for many people, but it isn't curative. And, like other physical modalities, it can aggravate chronic pain. If it helps generate more movement, better stretching, and an increase in activity, then it can be a useful technique in your arsenal of physical therapies. However, like massage therapy, it's a passive modality. Contrary to the belief of some, chiropractic manipulation is safe when practiced by a skilled clinician.

MYOFASCIAL RELEASE

Myofascial release is another hands-on muscle technique. It's based on the assumption that tight and restricted fascia, the connective tissue that covers the muscles, requires releasing. This technique is popular with many physical therapists, but again, it's a passive modality. It won't cure your chronic pain, but many of my patients testify that it helps them regain movement of their tight and deconditioned muscles.

HEAT AND COLD THERAPIES

Many people find temporary relief from muscle pain using heat and cold therapies. Heat can reduce muscle tension caused by stress, fatigue, or overused muscles. The heat is thought to increase blood flow to the muscles, raising oxygen levels and reducing chemical by-products that can irritate muscles. Cold can produce relief, too, by reducing inflammation and muscle spasm. Both heat and cold can be effective, but some people find more relief with one or the other.

All of the physical treatments discussed can provide temporary pain relief. You'll have to experiment to see which might help you. Keep in mind that none can cure chronic pain, but if they promote movement and relaxation of your muscles and help you to increase your activity level, they will help you manage your pain. However, remember that the best techniques are those you can apply yourself, without assistance, thereby decreasing your dependence on others.

Chemical Therapies

By far the most widely used biomedical treatments for pain are injections and medications. In addition to explaining different types of drugs, this section will discuss the concepts of tolerance, addiction, physical dependency, and withdrawal; the pros and cons of long-term management of chronic pain using narcotics; and various injection therapies.

MEDICATIONS FOR CHRONIC PAIN

In acute pain, medications are most often directed at the anatomic origin of pain, acting to reduce the cause of the pain. However, as chronic pain develops, the nature of pain transmission and reception changes, making it necessary to use drugs that can act at the source of pain but also treat the secondary complications of chronic pain, including emotional distress (Polatin and Gajraj 2002). The types of drugs most commonly prescribed for chronic pain are narcotics, nonnarcotic analgesics, antidepressants, anticonvulsants, tranquilizers, and muscle relaxers.

Before we examine each of these types of drugs, let's take a look at some confusing and controversial terms you need to understand: addiction, physical dependence, tolerance, and withdrawal. Many people, physicians and patients alike, make incorrect assumptions about these terms, and sometimes base their decisions about using different drugs on these assumptions.

Physical dependence refers to the body's adaptation to a drug and is characterized by the development of tolerance and the experience of withdrawal if the drug is stopped abruptly for a prolonged period (Fishbain, Rosomoff, and Rosomoff 1992). *Withdrawal* generally involves very uncomfortable physical symptoms, such as muscle cramping and diarrhea. *Tolerance* means having to take higher doses to achieve the effect of the drug, including pain relief, sedation, and euphoria. *Addiction* is compulsive use of a drug associated with cravings. It also implies misuse of the drug, such as taking narcotics for sedation and euphoria and not primarily for pain relief. Most importantly, addiction refers to continued use of a drug despite adverse social, health-related, economic, and occupational consequences.

NARCOTIC DRUGS

The type of medication most widely used to treat chronic pain is narcotics, also known as opioids. Narcotics are especially useful in the treatment of acute pain. They effectively relieve pain, often promote a general sense of relaxation, and can induce euphoria or a heightened sense of well-being. However, the use of narcotics in the treatment of chronic, nonmalignant pain isn't as widely endorsed by pain experts for several reasons: ineffectiveness, adverse effects, addiction, dependency, and the fact that they do little to address suffering.

Effectiveness. Although some people with chronic pain experience significant relief with narcotics, several studies question whether these drugs significantly ameliorate pain for most (Fishbain, Rosomoff, and Rosomoff 1992). In one of the few controlled studies examining the effects of narcotics for use with chronic pain patients, the authors reported that oral morphine provided only modest relief and no significant psychological or functional improvement (Moulin et al. 1996). In addition, patients receiving morphine reported other problems including vomiting (39 percent), dizziness (37 percent), constipation (41 percent), poor appetite or nausea (39 percent), and abdominal pain. The College of Physicians and Surgeons of Ontario (2000) reported that narcotics might be beneficial for short periods (nine weeks), but that long-term use doesn't appear to affect activity levels and other indicators of functional status. One well-controlled study examined differences between chronic pain patients taking narcotics versus those taking no narcotics. All patients participated in an outpatient rehabilitation pain program. All but 3 of 135 patients taking narcotics successfully discontinued their use by the end of the program, and there were no significant differences in measures of psychological distress and activity levels between the two groups.

Adverse effects.   Narcotics are associated with a number of problems, including compromised neuropsychological functioning (McNairy et al. 1984), gastrointestinal complaints such as constipation and vomiting (Rome et al. 2004), and a decline in sexual functioning and desire for sex (Ballantyne and Mao 2003). Recent investigations have also strongly suggested that narcotics may suppress the function of the immune system and important hormones (Ballantyne and Mao 2003). Interestingly, in the study of people in an outpatient rehabilitation pain program mentioned above (Rome et al. 2004), patients taking narcotics prior to participating in the program reported slightly higher pain intensities at the end even though there were no differences in pain severity between the two groups at the outset. The researchers concluded this might be due to either withdrawal or anxiety about coping without narcotics, or perhaps *hyperalgesia*, or increased pain, which is sometimes associated with chronic narcotic usage. This is thought to be a result of changes in the neurocircuitry of the spinal cord and brain.

Confounding pain with suffering. Physicians often observe patients suffering and assume pain is the sole cause of their misery. While unremitting pain is distressing and difficult to cope with, people also suffer because their chronic pain has turned their life upside down, causing financial problems, disturbed sleep, and marital difficulties, and interfering with day-to-day life. This type of suffering won't go away with a pill, and in fact, complications due to use of narcotics often compound people's problems.

Addiction. Many physicians only reluctantly prescribe narcotics to chronic pain patients out of concerns about addiction. Mistakenly assuming the amount of the drug sets the stage for addiction, they place patients on as-needed dosing and prescribe inadequate amounts or stretch the intervals between doses. However, these tactics actually increase susceptibility to addiction, as it results in people waiting until they have high levels of pain before taking a pill and then often taking more than they need because the pain level is so distressing. When the drug finally takes effect, its use is reinforced both psychologically and physically. In fact, the incidence of addiction to narcotics is actually very low in people with chronic pain (Fishbain, Rosomoff, and Rosomoff 1992). Reluctance to prescribe narcotics should not be from a fear of addiction. But keep in mind that there are many other good reasons, mentioned above, for not taking them.

Dependency. Another problem with taking narcotics is that they can foster a dependency on something outside yourself. When you think, "It's the drug and not me that's making a difference in my pain," it reduces your sense of personal control. Narcotics can also prevent you from turning your efforts to more active and sustainable pain management strategies, such as pacing. People taking narcotics often forgo limiting their activities to achievable levels because they know they can rescue themselves with a pill. This is ultimately self-defeating, leading to a boom-and-bust cycle, escalating fears of pain, and, in the end, reduced levels of activity.

Some people with chronic pain can, in fact, do well taking narcotics on a long-term basis, but they are in the minority. Candidates for long-term use must fulfill a long list of qualifications: They don't experience significant adverse side effects. They can honestly say that they receive more than 20 percent relief from narcotics. They are significantly more active when taking narcotics. They don't escalate their dose. And their use of the drug isn't an avoidance strategy, allowing them to mitigate their fear of pain.

NONNARCOTIC ANALGESICS

Nonnarcotic analgesics include acetaminophen (for example, Tylenol), aspirin, and the nonsteroidal anti-inflammatory drugs (NSAIDs), such as ibuprofen. The NSAIDs are generally most effective in pain conditions where there's a proven inflammatory process, such as osteoarthritis and rheumatoid arthritis. Beyond that, they're of only limited use in chronic pain, where in so many cases the original injury and any inflammation have long since resolved.

Side effects, especially irritation of the stomach, colon, and esophagus, are common with nonsteroidal anti-inflammatory drugs. They can also damage the liver and kidneys, increase bleeding time and sensitivity to bruising, and cause rashes, tinnitus, and sensitivity to light (Polatin and Gajraj 2002). Physical dependency and addiction don't occur with nonnarcotic analgesics.

If you're taking nonnarcotic analgesics, ask your doctor whether they're genuinely necessary. And if you're taking an NSAID, ask whether you should undergo periodic testing of your liver function. If you aren't sure if a nonnarcotic analgesic is helping you, consider a holiday from the drug to determine if it's truly beneficial, but only after consultation with your doctor.

ANTIDEPRESSANTS

Antidepressants have been used in the management of pain for quite some time. They've been shown to alleviate headaches and certain types of nerve pain known as *neuropathic pain*. They're less effective in treating low back pain and arthritis (Polatin and Gajraj 2002). It appears that they truly provide relief from pain.

Although all antidepressants have been shown to have some analgesic benefit, including the new ones such as Prozac (fluoxetine), some are more effective in reducing pain, especially neuropathic pain and headache pain (Polatin and Gajraj 2002). Falling into a class known as tricyclic antidepressants, these include Elavil (amitriptyline), Norpramin (desipramine), Sinequan (doxepin), Tofranil (imipramine), and Anafranil (clomipramine). Their increased efficacy is believed to result from their ability to block reuptake of the neurochemical norepinephrine, not just serotonin. This is also true for a newer class of antidepressants called dual uptake inhibitors (for example, Cymbalta, or duloxetine). These drugs act very much like tricyclic antidepressants.

Tricyclic antidepressants and dual uptake inhibitors can cause significant sedation, so they're also often used to facilitate sleep and prescribed at bedtime. However, even very low doses can cause some people to feel tired and hungover the next day. Most people, but not all, eventually adapt and have increased tolerance in regard to sedation. If you decide to take an antidepressant, it's important to start at a low dose and gradually increase it until you experience optimal pain relief with a minimum of uncomfortable side effects, which may include dry mouth, blurry vision, and, for some people, increased appetite leading to weight gain. Antidepressants aren't associated with physical dependency and addiction.

ANTICONVULSANTS

Anticonvulsants are thought to inhibit the excitatory properties of nerves, thereby stabilizing nerve membranes. They've been shown to be particularly effective in treating pain conditions associated with diabetes, neuropathy, migraine headaches, and certain forms of neuralgia. A newer class of anticonvulsants, including Neurontin (gabapentin), Topamax (topiramate), and Lyrica (pregabalin), tends to be better tolerated by patients, but they're still associated with sedation, dizziness, and spaciness. They can also cause gastrointestinal symptoms in some patients. An older anticonvulsant, Klonopin (clonazepam), is often prescribed because it's also a benzodiazepine tranquilizer, but for that very same reason, it carries some risk of addiction and physical dependence. As with antidepressants, it's best to start with a low dose and gradually increase the amount taken to find what level produces the most benefits while minimizing side effects.

TRANQUILIZERS

Tranquilizers or antianxiety medications, such as Xanax (alprazolam), Valium (diazepam), Klonopin (clonazepam), BuSpar (buspirone), and Ativan (lorazepam), are often prescribed for the anxiety symptoms that can occur with chronic pain (which can increase pain perception and disrupt coping mechanisms). Although they can be useful as short-term treatments for reducing anxiety and muscle tension, they don't appear to be useful long-term tools for managing chronic pain. Klonopin may be the exception because, as an anticonvulsant, it's used to treat neuropathic pain.

Most tranquilizers can cause physical dependency and addiction and have side effects that include sedation, drowsiness, and confusion. Many physicians also prescribe tranquilizers to help with sleep problems, but they aren't effective in aiding sleep for more than a few weeks; plus, they disrupt deep sleep and REM sleep and can lead to physical dependency.

MUSCLE RELAXERS

Muscle relaxers, also known as antispasmodics, help relax skeletal muscles and have effects similar to benzodiazepines, or tranquilizers. Although considered to have some use in treating transient or acute pain, they're generally of little therapeutic value in treating chronic pain (Schoefferman 1994) with the exception of Lioresal (baclofen), which is effective in a few specific chronic pain conditions. Many muscle relaxers, especially Soma (carisoprodol), are associated with physical dependency and addiction and all of them can cause excessive sedation. They may disrupt deep sleep and REM sleep, and when they wear off, they can cause rebound muscle spasm.

INJECTION THERAPIES

Chemicals can also be delivered by injection. It's a fairly common practice to use joint, bursa, and epidural injections of steroids and other agents, alone or in combination, to reduce pain. Though these therapies can provide substantial pain relief, their effect is usually short-lived. It can be considered useful to the extent that the relief it provides stimulates movement and general activity.

IMPLANTED MORPHINE PUMPS

The morphine pump, or intrathecal pump, delivers morphine and other drugs using an implantable catheter. This device is considered a useful alternative for patients taking high oral doses of narcotics since the delivery mechanism is superior to oral dosing or injections. It is, however, an extreme measure for most patients since it carries the risk of complications, including nerve damage, infection, and dislodgement of the catheter. It is also associated with uncomfortable side effects, especially nausea and vomiting, sedation, and itching.

Newer studies have linked long-term use of a morphine pump to depletion of growth hormone, gonadal hormones, and corticosteroids, which usually leads to decreased libido and irregular menstrual cycles, among other problems (Abs et al. 2000). Despite the potential for severe complications and side effects, for some people the morphine pump can be very effective for relieving intractable, noncancerous pain. However, most studies examining their effectiveness have been of poor quality, making it difficult to draw definitive conclusions.

Electrical Therapies

Electrical interventions attempt to disrupt, or "scramble," the pain signal as it travels to the spinal cord and brain, causing a reduction in pain or reception of a signal that is interpreted as nonpainful. Based on the gate control theory discussed in chapter 1, the use of electrical devices for treating pain is well established.

TRANSCUTANEOUS ELECTRICAL NERVE STIMULATION

Although there are many forms of electrical treatment, the most widely used external method is transcutaneous electrical nerve stimulation (TENS). Adhesive pads are placed over localized areas of pain. Wires are attached to the pads and an external device is used to generate a mild electrical signal. TENS has been shown to be useful in a significant minority of people with chronic pain. However, the vast majority of studies of TENS indicate it's premature to make any firm conclusions about its general and long-term effectiveness and the parameters that should be used for different pain conditions (Carroll et al. 2001).

IMPLANTABLE ELECTRICAL NERVE STIMULATION

In the past decade, implantable electric stimulators have been used to treat intractable pain. Initially used to apply electrical stimulation to the dorsal columns of the spinal cord (Shealy, Mortimer, and Rewick 1967), it has become increasingly popular for treating a variety of pain syndromes.

Spinal cord stimulation involves the insertion of electrodes under local anesthesia. The electrodes are placed at the appropriate position on the spine to achieve maximum benefit. The electrodes are attached to an internally placed electrical stimulator to generate an electrical signal, and the patient can control the amount and duration of stimulation.

Spinal cord stimulation has been shown to be useful in a variety of intractable pain conditions, especially complex regional pain syndrome (which some still refer to as reflex sympathetic dystrophy), postamputation pain, postherpetic neuralgia, spinal cord injury, dysesthesias, and pain related to multiple sclerosis (Gatchel 2005).

Surgical Treatments

Surgery can be helpful for alleviating many types of acute pain, but it's much less successful in treating chronic pain. One reason is because the underlying pain mechanism is unclear in most people with chronic pain, especially those with low back pain. The many secondary problems that develop over time, such as musculoskeletal pain and psychological distress, cloud the picture further. Studies have consistently shown that the chances of a second operation succeeding when the first has failed are low—and lower still for any subsequent operation.

Sometimes surgery is a necessity, but not often. Make sure you seek a second opinion and even a third if it will make you more confident about what could be a life-altering decision. Consider seeking additional opinions from a nonsurgical pain specialist, who will be more likely to view surgery as just one of several therapeutic options.

Biomedical treatments for pain can be very effective in the management of chronic pain. Although not curative, they can decrease pain intensity and promote increased activity, which is beneficial in many ways, particularly for musculoskeletal health. The effectiveness of biomedical treatments for chronic pain is enhanced when they're combined with behavioral and psychological interventions. This includes attention to how others can influence your pain and disability. This is the topic of chapter 10, the last solution to managing your chronic pain.

10 Recognizing the Influence of Others

For years, psychologists have recognized that social factors can exert a tremendous influence on pain and disability. This chapter explores how this dynamic works and will teach you how to lessen the negative impacts of your chronic pain by relating to others more effectively, particularly in regard to your pain.

■ Glen's Story

Glen developed chronic neck pain after he rolled his pickup. During his recovery, his wife helped him dress and bathe. She brought his meals to him in bed and massaged his tight shoulder muscles. Glen said he wouldn't have been able to get along without her.

Eight weeks after his accident, Glen still hadn't returned to work. His pain was worse and his sleep was restless. Glen's wife worried about him. She didn't understand why he wasn't improving and

*was frustrated with his doctors. She was convinced
they weren't doing enough to help him. She watched
Glen like a hawk, making sure he was comfortable,
especially when she could tell he was having a bad
day. She also warned him not to pick up things or
push himself too hard, and when he did, she gave
him a look that said, "I told you so."*

*Glen liked the fact that his wife cared so much,
but after several months in pain he occasionally
snapped at her when she babied him too much. He
sometimes wondered if she was growing tired of
him, and he felt guilty for flying off the handle and
burdening her with his misery. He started to spend
more time in his room when his pain flared up,
worried he would lose his temper in her presence.
When asked if he thought his marriage was good,
Glen said, "The best. I couldn't ask for a better wife.
I don't know how she puts up with me."*

Pain and Your Life Partner

Several years ago, Dr. Michael Lewandowski and I collected
information from several hundred chronic pain patients about
their spouses (Tearnan and Lewandowski 1992). We were inter-
ested in how patients described what their spouse did when
they showed pain behaviors or wellness behaviors. We wanted
to see if the spouse's behavior in any way affected the patient's
perceived level of disability. We defined *pain behaviors* as those
things people do when they're in pain to communicate to others
that they're suffering; examples include groaning, moaning,
walking with a limp, asking for pain medications, crying, and
becoming quiet. *Wellness behaviors* are things people do to show
others they're active and not sick or suffering.

We also looked at whether the patients reported that their spouse reacted negatively or positively to their pain or wellness behavior. For example, a positive response to pain behavior would be giving the person a back rub. A negative response would be criticizing the person for not doing more. A positive response to wellness would be praising the person for being up and active. A negative response would be warning or discouraging the person from lifting or other activities. Our survey confirmed our clinical observations, which you may find surprising. Disability levels tend to increase whether spouses show positive or negative responses to either pain or wellness behaviors. The main differences between these categories are degree of disability. Let's take a closer look at each of the four types of interactions and its effect on disability.

POSITIVE RESPONSE TO PAIN BEHAVIOR

Positive responses to pain behaviors include paying more attention when the person appears to be in pain, waiting on them when they say they hurt, and giving back rubs in response to increased complaints of pain. Patients who said their spouse showed positive responses to their pain behaviors reported higher levels of disability. This tends to happen because positive reinforcement affects behavior. If your spouse is more attentive or positive when you exhibit pain behavior, there's a good chance you'll exhibit such behaviors more frequently, often without any awareness on your part.

In Glen's case, his wife did everything for him. She listened to his complaints and went out of her way to comfort him. For the most part, Glen enjoyed this, and in some ways he felt closer to her after his injury. However, her behavior also increased Glen's dependence on her and subtly changed his perception of himself. He no longer felt as confident and sure of himself and often turned to her for assistance, even for doing things he could manage on his own.

The dynamics of the relationship also started to change. Before Glen's injury, he and his wife would talk about all sorts of things, but afterward their conversation seemed to be centered on how he was feeling. They also started to express their affection differently, with a focus on concern and caring about Glen's condition: "How are you feeling, sweetie? Can I get you something?" The real danger for Glen was that he had assumed the role of a sick person in relation to his wife. He was a patient and she was his nurse. He was passive and dependent on her and had lost confidence in his ability to cope.

NEGATIVE RESPONSE TO WELLNESS BEHAVIOR

Negative responses to wellness behavior can have effects on disability that are very similar to the effects of a positive response to pain behaviors, such as increased dependency and illness behavior. Frequent admonitions by others about the negative consequences of activity can also strengthen fears of reinjury, leading to increased avoidance behavior.

NEGATIVE RESPONSE TO PAIN BEHAVIOR

The strongest association between spousal behavior and increased disability occurred when spouses responded negatively to pain behavior. In this case, patients were also much more likely to be angry, depressed, and dissatisfied with their medical care. The patients said this response showed that their spouse didn't care and didn't think their pain was legitimate. Disability probably increased because the patients wanted to show their spouse that their pain was legitimate. These patients were also much more likely to be depressed, which can also contribute to higher levels of disability.

When we interviewed spouses who showed a negative response to pain behavior, they often revealed resentful feelings and disbelief about the seriousness of their spouse's pain. Ignorance about chronic pain was at the core of why they responded the way they did. Almost without exception, patients described their marriage as unhappy if they felt their spouse responded negatively to their pain.

POSITIVE RESPONSE TO WELLNESS BEHAVIOR

We were somewhat surprised to find that a positive response to wellness behaviors wasn't strongly associated with an increase in reported wellness behaviors. In fact, many patients in this situation had increased levels of disability. This seems to go against common sense and what we know about positive reinforcement, but it turned out that the reason was similar to what we found in patients whose spouses showed negative responses to pain behavior: If their spouse didn't respond to their pain beyond encouraging them to increase their activities, patients often felt resentful and interpreted their spouse's behavior as uncaring and unsympathetic. Again, many patients seemed to respond by trying, usually unintentionally, to prove their pain was legitimate by increasing their levels of disability.

However, if their spouse was attentive to their pain behavior and attempted to discourage their efforts to engage in certain activities, patients concluded that their spouse cared for them. And when their spouse showed a high positive response to pain behavior and a negative response to wellness, patients generally reported increased marital satisfaction.

TECHNIQUES FOR IMPROVING YOUR INTERACTIONS WITH OTHERS

The four types of interactions described above also apply to your relationships with your friends and others, not just your spouse or significant other. At first, it might be hard for you to recognize that others can impact your behavior so strongly. Most of us resist the idea that we don't have complete control of our behavior and that we're subject to influences outside of ourselves. However, try to be open to the possibility while keeping in mind that social influences are just one factor in how you think and behave in relation to your pain. However, since relationships can have a huge impact on mood and quality of life, you'll probably find it highly rewarding to work on this issue using the techniques presented below.

To change your interactions with others, you'll have to recognize that it's up to you to initiate any changes you want. Your spouse, boyfriend or girlfriend, friends, and family, and even your doctors, are unlikely to alter their behavior if you don't make some changes first. Some people might resist change at first, since the consequences of their behavior may be highly reinforcing for them. For example, a husband who's overly attentive might believe his efforts are keeping his wife safe from harm. He might also think it's an expression of his love to wait on her and ease her suffering, thereby fulfilling his role as a protector and caring husband.

Also bear in mind that you only have so much control over how others behave toward you. This doesn't mean, however, that you can't reduce the impact of your interactions. Another potential problem is that you might be reluctant to give up the attention and caring expressed by others. You have to take a close look and decide what's best for you and your relationships. Again, be open and honest in your analysis of how others may be impacting your behavior and in turn your levels of disability.

Exercise: Learning More About Your Interactions

By now you have a better idea of how others might be affecting your level of disability. This exercise will help you further clarify the nature of your interactions. For each statement below, select the one answer that best describes how much you agree or disagree with the statement. For example, if you strongly agree with an item, answer 5, 6, or 7. If you strongly disagree with an item, answer 0, 1, or 2. If you moderately agree or feel neutral about an item, answer 3 or 4.

```
0    1    2    3    4    5    6    7
Strongly disagree      Strongly agree
```

PAIN BEHAVIOR: POSITIVE RESPONSE

1. People tend to pay more attention to my needs when I'm in pain than when I'm not. _____

2. People encourage me to rest when I'm in pain. _____

3. People are especially nice to me when I'm in pain. _____

4. People often ask how I feel when I'm in pain. _____

PAIN BEHAVIOR: NEGATIVE RESPONSE

1. People complain that my pain has made their life difficult. _____

2. People get irritated and angry
   at me because of my pain.   _____

3. People get irritated with me
   for not getting better.   _____

4. People get mad at me when
   I tell them I'm in pain.   _____

WELLNESS BEHAVIOR: POSITIVE RESPONSE

1. People encourage me to do my
   chores and duties.   _____

2. People tell me they like it when
   I increase my physical activity. _____

3. People pay attention to me when
   I'm physically active—for
   example, doing chores.   _____

WELLNESS BEHAVIOR: NEGATIVE RESPONSE

1. People become irritated with
   me when I try to increase my
   physical activity.   _____

2. People often caution me about
   reinjuring myself when I'm
   physically active.   _____

3. When I'm active, people often
   warn me, "You'll pay the price
   if you keep that up."   _____

Tally your scores for each type of interaction, then divide by the number of questions to calculate your average score for each category. A score of 4 or above for any of these types of interactions indicates a strong likelihood this type of dynamic may be operating in your relationships.

CHALLENGE BELIEFS ABOUT RELATIONSHIPS

Changing the way you interact with others in relation to your pain is difficult, and you may resist. This may be due to nonproductive beliefs about your relationships, in which case it's important to challenge these beliefs before moving forward. Otherwise, you may undermine your efforts to successfully change your interactions with others.

Exercise: Challenging Beliefs That Can Interfere with Change

For each statement below, ask yourself if you think the belief is true. For those you believe to be true, practice challenging them using the skills you learned in chapter 5.

- If others stop paying attention to my pain behavior or stop discouraging me from doing certain things, it would mean they don't care about me.

- If others stop paying attention to my pain behavior or stop discouraging me from doing certain things, I would be all alone.

- If I changed the way others respond to me, they would expect too much of me.

- I'm too helpless to let go of the attention I receive because of my pain.

- I'm not sure I would know what to do if others treated me as healthy and not sick.

ADDRESS OTHERS' BELIEFS AND MISPERCEPTIONS ABOUT YOUR PAIN

It's important that, at some point, you sit down and talk with others close to you about your pain and how it has affected your life and theirs. Although this will be difficult, it will also be helpful, clearing the air and allowing everyone to talk about their frustrations, their fears, and any feelings of resentment. People in pain often want to sweep the discussion of problems under the rug to avoid stirring up hurtful feelings, but silence leaves everyone pretending nothing's wrong. There's no shame in the problems that have beset you since pain started to dominate your life. You're struggling with difficulties every person in chronic pain confronts. Talking with your family and friends about these issues will help them feel closer to you and reduce their sense of helplessness, especially if they often try to, or have to, second-guess what is bothering you.

A good starting point is to let others know you're ready to move on with your life—that you've waited long enough for the elusive cure and now you want to move forward. Reassure them that you're healthy in spite of certain limitations and that chronic pain is not a sentence of doom. Challenge their desire to keep on searching for a cure, and remind them that your doctors have told you that you have a stable medical condition and need no further aggressive care. If your doctor is planning additional treatment, tell your family and friends what the short- and long-term goals are, and that your pursuit of treatments doesn't mean your life should remain on hold.

Ask others what they fear about your pain. What is their biggest fear? Reinjury? A setback in your healing? Reassure them by giving them the facts, data, and proof that you are okay.

It's also important to tell others that you want to take care of your own needs. Acknowledge that you appreciate their help and support, then explain why it's important that you start to do more for yourself. If they seem disappointed, explain that you still very much need their affection and love, just not directed at your pain.

Understanding others' perspective about you since the onset of your pain is also vital. How do they think you've changed as a person? Do they see you as weak and frail, or strong with certain limitations? What things about you tell them you're different? Are their perceptions accurate? What would you need to change or what would have to happen for them to see you differently?

There's no exact script to follow in your discussions with others; the suggestions above are simply designed to stimulate your thoughts and give you some guidance. Try to be flexible and remember that hurt or angry feelings might surface. Try to work through these and be prepared to take a break and try again if conversations get stalled or too heated. The important thing is that you're talking, and this presents you with more opportunities than ignoring your problems.

Exercise: Magnifying Pain Behavior

This exercise is useful for stimulating ideas for your discussions with others. When you're with family or friends, magnify your pain behavior. If you normally ask for help, grimace, or walk with a distorted gait, intensify these behaviors. The purpose is to see how your family and friends respond to you. After a couple of minutes, let them know what you're doing and why. Ask them the following questions:

- What did you think when you saw me hurting?

- Did you feel sorry for me? About what?

- Were you worried? About what?

- Were you frustrated? About what?

- What did you think you had to do to comfort me?

Explore as much as you can any thoughts and feelings your friends and family had, as well as any desires to leave you alone. How did their responses tie in with your thoughts about the four types of interactions described earlier?

BREAKING PATTERNS

The preceding exercises and techniques have probably given you some good ideas about the nature of your interactions with others in relation to your pain. To change any problematic patterns, you need to redefine the way others relate to you when you're in pain. Ideally, you want to deemphasize pain and have others reinforce your wellness behaviors. Here are some techniques that will help you accomplish this:

- Remind others to express their love and affection in ways other than showing sympathy and caring for your needs in relation to your pain. There are many other ways they can be affectionate with you.

- Resist others' efforts to take over and protect you. Reassure them often that you won't break in two when you start to resume your activities. Be assertive when you tell them not to warn you against attempts to be active, even if your pain increases.

- Try to ignore any criticisms you hear about your pain, but do sit down with people who do this and try to understand their thoughts. If you're too uncomfortable doing this, you may need help from a family member, friend, or a trusted professional.

- Take a less passive role in your relations with others. Tell them your needs and take action to make these things happen. Suggest activities to do together, and if they resist because of your pain, gently remind them that you're setting your own limitations but appreciate their concern.

- Establish activities you can do separately from your family, friends, and spouse. This will help build your confidence that you can be self-reliant and show others you don't always need their watchful eye. Start small and gradually increase the amount of time and distance you're away from them. Make your excursions fun.

- It's important to share with others what you're learning about pain. Tell them what your quotas are and how you established them. Talk about the nature of chronic pain and encourage them to read this book. Help them see pain as less mysterious, just as you have. This will help them feel more comfortable letting go of the responsibility for looking out for you.

LEARN TO BE A COUPLE AGAIN

It's important to think of things you and your spouse or significant other can do to bring more fun and romance to your relationship. When one partner is in pain, the relationship may become dominated by attempts to prevent, minimize, or control the pain. Rewarding aspects of the relationship are often put on hold as you both wait for the pain to go away. You may have stopped going out together, having sex, getting together with friends, or traveling. Pain may restrict certain activities, but it's important that you figure out fun things you can do that are within your limitations. Set a goal of going out to a restaurant or some other type of entertainment. If your ability to sit is limited, work on increasing your tolerance first before venturing out.

Try to put more romance in your relationship, including increasing the frequency of sex. If sex increases your pain, explore different positions and learn to be more open with each other about what feels good that doesn't cause your pain to flare up. A decline in sexual functioning is common with chronic pain, and isn't solely due to the pain. Many medications, particularly narcotics, can decrease the desire for sex and disrupt performance. Fatigue, anxiety, and strain in your relationship can also hinder normal sexual relations. If open and honest discussions with your partner don't improve things, explore the problem with your doctor to see whether any physical factors are affecting your sex life, and if needed, ask for a referral to a mental health professional specializing in pain.

Improving Your Relationships with Your Doctors

Knowing how to develop a good patient-doctor relationship is especially important for people in chronic pain, since this relationship is frequently strained for many reasons. The biggest reason is that your pain hasn't responded to conventional medical care, so your doctor may feel frustrated, defeated, and unsure what to do next. Doctors want to see results, and it's tough to face the fact that your pain hasn't gone away. A good relationship with your doctor will ensure that you're satisfied with your care and better able to accept the decisions you and your doctor make together. It also helps you have a higher level of trust in your doctor and greater overall confidence.

Improving your relationships with your doctors involves decreasing your passivity and increasing your active involvement in your care. If you're more involved, you'll have an increased sense of personal control and mastery in managing your pain. You'll also be less likely to rely on your doctor and adopt a sick role, which will boost your confidence about managing pain on your own.

Your doctor's attitude is important in creating this sort of relationship. It's immensely helpful if your doctor encourages self-responsibility and is careful not to foster dependency.

Doctors with this orientation understand that coping with chronic pain can be a rough process, but they gently encourage patients to increase their activity level and are reluctant to use narcotics in high doses. They don't always give patients what they want, but they are willing to discuss their reasons for saying no. Your doctor should provide guidelines on what activities you can do, how to do them safely, and how you can manage your pain better. One of the most important things a doctor can do is to educate you to help reduce your fears. A doctor should be a healer and teacher.

TIPS FOR IMPROVING YOUR RELATIONSHIPS WITH YOUR DOCTORS

With all you've been through, you may believe that there's little you can do to change your relationship with your doctors and that it's the luck of the draw as to whether a good relationship develops. Fortunately, this is not the case. You can use the techniques described below to improve your relationship and get the most out of your interactions with your doctors.

CLARIFY YOUR EXPECTATIONS

Take some time to seriously consider what you want out of your relationship with your doctor. Be realistic. Doctors can only do so much, and often that's very little when it comes to helping you manage chronic pain. They can help clarify aspects of your medical condition, educate you, and administer certain treatments such as medications, but they can't cure you or significantly reduce your pain. They can't always rescue you, and they're unlikely to counsel you about your psychological needs, but if you have a good relationship, your doctor will guide you.

CLARIFY YOUR DOCTOR'S EXPECTATIONS

What are your responsibilities as a patient, and what does your doctor expect from you? For example, how does your doctor want you to manage your flare-ups if you run out of medications prematurely? Can you call the office between appointments, and whom should you speak with if your doctor isn't available? What is your doctor's philosophy of treatment, and what does he or she consider to be a successful outcome? Ask any questions necessary to clarify your doctor's expectations.

ASK THE RIGHT KINDS OF QUESTIONS

Uncertainty about your medical status can contribute to anxiety and make you feel that you aren't in control of your situation. Keep track of any questions you have about your medical status so that you'll remember everything you want to ask when you visit your doctor. Be assertive. Most doctors will listen, respect your desire to know, and do their best to answer each question, but you have to remember to ask them! If necessary, review chapter 3 for guidance on the kinds of information that will be most helpful to you.

EXPECT PROBLEMS

No relationship is perfect, and this seems to be especially true with doctors, in part because there's almost always some stress involved in seeing a doctor. At times you may feel overwhelmed, confused, angry, and disappointed. Remember that a certain amount of conflict is inevitable and that you'll sometimes hit rough spots. This is usually due to a failure to clarify expectations and to communicate your needs. Doctors aren't mind readers, and they can't help you as effectively if you aren't forthcoming about your symptoms, concerns, fears, and frustrations.

ASSUME SELF-RESPONSIBILITY

Your relationship with your doctor will be much stronger when you take charge and accept responsibility for making changes. Ultimately, successful management of your pain isn't up to your doctor, it's up to you. Your doctor can guide you, but you have to make the hard choices and commit to changing your lifestyle. If you accept this, you won't expect so much from your doctor and be disappointed when he or she falls short of your expectations. You won't feel as helpless and as a result will turn confidently to yourself for the answers you need.

Our relationships have a great impact on our feelings of well-being, whether or not we're dealing with chronic pain. Though there's much you can do on your own to improve your experience of pain and quality of life, for the greatest long-term success you also need to have healthy relationships—particularly in regard to your pain. Using the exercises and techniques you've learned in this chapter will ensure that your relationships support all of the solutions this book has offered.

Afterword

Many of the changes that will help you better manage and cope with your chronic pain will need to be practiced for a long time. This isn't an easy task, but it isn't impossible. You've learned the skills, and now it's time to practice what you've learned. You may need to reread some or all of the chapters from time to time to refresh your memory and deepen your understanding of the material in this book. Using the behavior change strategies discussed in chapter 2, develop a daily game plan and stick with it. Practice until you're comfortable and confident with your daily routine, making adjustments as necessary to fit your needs. Do whatever is necessary to make things work and to keep yourself moving forward.

Expect to stumble at times. If you don't, you aren't taking the risks necessary to succeed in the long term. Learn to anticipate likely problems as you journey forward. How will you handle future flare-ups? What if you feel overwhelmed with problems again? How would you work your way through them? When might you need help, and where will you turn to find it? If you lose interest in practicing your daily routine, how will you stay motivated about following through on your program?

Make it a habit to periodically take the BAPSI assessment in chapter 4. Are you satisfied with your current levels of functioning and mood? What areas do you need to focus on so you can maintain the gains you've made? Are there other goals you'd like to work on?

Congratulations on finishing the book. I know you still have work to do and that there are things you didn't accomplish to the degree you wanted, but this is to be expected. You'll learn to better apply the skills in this book with time and effort. However, for now, pat yourself on the back and be assured that you have the basic tools to move forward with your life despite your pain—a life of hope and promise.

Recommended Readings

Anderson, N. B., and P. E. Anderson. 2003. *Emotional Longevity*. New York: Viking.

Benson, H. 1976. *The Relaxation Response*. New York: William Morrow.

Benson, H., and E. Stuart. 1993. *The Wellness Book: The Comprehensive Guide to Maintaining Health and Treating Stress-Related Illness*. Secaucus, NJ: Birch Lane Press.

Burns, D. D. 1999. *The Feeling Good Handbook*. New York: Plume.

Gatchel, R. J. 2005. *Clinical Essentials of Pain Management*. Washington, DC: American Psychological Association.

Hage, M. 1992. *The Back Pain Book*. Atlanta, GA: Peachtree Publishers.

Jacobs, G. D. 1998. *Say Good Night to Insomnia*. New York: Henry Holt.

Kabat-Zinn, J. 1990. *Full Catastrophe Living.* New York: Delta Books.

Lycholat, T. 1995. *The Complete Book of Stretching.* Ramsbury Marlborough, England: Crowood.

Marcus, D. A. 2006. *10 Simple Solutions to Migraines.* Oakland, CA: New Harbinger Publications.

Starlanyl, D., and M. E. Copeland. 2001. *Fibromyalgia and Chronic Myofascial Pain: A Survival Manual.* Oakland, CA: New Harbinger Publications.

Thorn, B. E. 2004. *Cognitive Therapy for Chronic Pain.* New York: Guilford Press.

Wilson, A. 1994. *Are You Sitting Comfortably? A Self-Help Guide for Sufferers of Back Pain, Neck Strain, Headaches, RSI, and Other Health Problems.* London: Optima.

References

Abs, R., J. Verhelst, J. Maeyaert, J. Van Buyten, F. Opsomer, H. Adriaensen, J. Verlooy, T. Van Havenbergh, M. Smet, and K. Van Acker. 2000. Endocrine consequences of long-term intrathecal administration of opioids. *Journal of Clinical Endocrinology and Metabolism* 85(6):2215-2222.

Anderson, N. B., and P. E. Anderson. 2003. *Emotional Longevity*. New York: Viking.

Antony, M. M., and R. E. McCabe. 2004. *10 Simple Solutions to Panic*. Oakland, CA: New Harbinger Publications.

Asmundson, G. J. 1999. Anxiety sensitivity and chronic pain: Empirical findings, clinical implications, and future directions. In *Anxiety Sensitivity: Theory, Research, and Treatment of the Fear of Anxiety*, ed. S. Taylor, 269-285. London: Lawrence Erlbaum Associates.

Ballantyne, J. C., and J. Mao. 2003. Opioid therapy for chronic pain. *New England Journal of Medicine* 349(20):1943-1953.

Beck, A., J. Rush, B. Shaw, and G. Emery. 1979. *Cognitive Therapy for Depression*. New York: Guilford Press.

Burns, D. D. 1999. *The Feeling Good Handbook*. New York: Plume.

Carroll, D., R. A. Moore, H. J. McQuay, F. Fairman, M. Tramer, and G. Leijon. 2001. Transcutaneous electrical nerve stimulation (TENS) for chronic pain. *Cochrane Database of Systematic Reviews* 3:CD003222.

Cassell, E. J. 1982. The nature of suffering and the goals of medicine. *New England Journal of Medicine* 306(11):639-645.

College of Physicians and Surgeons of Ontario. 2000. *Evidence-Based Recommendations for Medical Management of Chronic Non-Malignant Pain: Reference Guide for Physicians*. Toronto: College of Physicians and Surgeons of Ontario.

Craig, K. D. 1994. Emotional aspects of pain. In *The Textbook of Pain*, ed. P. D. Wall and R. Melzack, 261-274. Edinburgh: Churchill Livingstone.

Dement, W. C. 1999. *The Promise of Sleep*. New York: Dell Trade.

Engel, G. L. 1977. The need for a new medical model: A challenge for biomedicine. *Science* 196(4286):129-136.

Fernandez, E., and D. C. Turk. 1995. The scope and significance of anger in the experience of chronic pain. *Pain* 61(2):165-175.

Fishbain, D. A., M. Goldberg, B. Meagher, R. Steele, and H. L. Rosomoff. 1986. Male and female chronic pain patients categorized by DSM-III psychiatric diagnostic criteria. *Pain* 26(2):181-197.

Fishbain, D. A., H. L. Rosomoff, and R. S. Rosomoff. 1992. Drug abuse, dependence, and addiction in chronic pain patients. *Clinical Journal of Pain* 8(2):77-85.

Fordyce, W. E. 1988. Pain and suffering: A reappraisal. *American Psychologist* 43(4):276-283.

Gatchel, R. J. 2005. *Clinical Essentials of Pain Management.* Washington, DC: American Psychological Association.

Gatchel, R. J., and D. C. Turk. 1996. *Psychological Approaches to Pain Management: A Practitioner's Handbook.* New York: Guilford Press.

Greenberger, D., and C. Padesky. 1990. *Cognitive Therapy: A Skills Building Workbook.* Unpublished.

Hafen, B. Q., K. J. Karren, K. J. Frandsen, and N. L. Smith. 1996. *Mind/Body Health: The Effects of Attitudes, Emotions, and Relationships.* Boston: Allyn and Bacon.

Hauri, P., and S. Linde. 1996. *No More Sleepless Nights.* New York: Wiley.

Holbrook, T. L., K. Grazier, J. L. Kelsey, and R. N. Stauffer. 1984. *The Frequency, Occurrence, Impact and Cost of Selected Musculoskeletal Conditions in the United States.* Park Ridge, IL: American Academy of Orthopedic Surgeons.

Jacobs, G. D. 1998. *Say Good Night to Insomnia.* New York: Henry Holt.

Kerns, R. D., R. Rosenberg, and M. C. Jacob. 1994. Anger expression and chronic pain. *Journal of Behavioral Medicine* 17(1):57-67.

Lazarus, R. S. 1994. *Emotion and Adaptation.* Cary, NC: Oxford University Press.

Leventhal, H., and D. Everhart. 1979. Emotion, pain, and physical illness. In *Emotion and Psychopathology*, ed. C. E. Izard, 263-299. New York: Plenum Press.

Loeser, J. D. 1982. Concepts of pain. In *Chronic Low Back Pain*, ed. J. Stanton-Hicks and R. Boaz, 109-142. New York: Raven Press.

McCracken, I. M., C. Zayfert, and R. T. Gross. 1993. The Pain Anxiety Symptom Scale (PASS): A multimodal measure of pain-specific anxiety symptoms. *Behavior Therapist* 16:183-184.

McNairy, S. L., T. Maruta, R. J. Ivnik, D. W. Swanson, and D. M. Ilstrup. 1984. Prescription medication dependence and neuropsychologic function. *Pain* 18(2):169-177.

Melzack, R., and P. D. Wall. 1965. Pain mechanisms: A new theory. *Science* 150(699):971-979.

Moulin, D. E., A. Iezzi, R. Amireh, W. K. Sharpe, D. Boyd, and H. Merskey. 1996. Randomised trial of oral morphine for chronic non-cancer pain. *Lancet* 347(8995):143-147.

Polatin, P. B., and N. M. Gajraj. 2002. Integration of pharmacotherapy with psychological treatment of chronic pain. In *Psychological Approaches to Pain Management: A Practitioner's Handbook*, ed. D. C. Turk and R. J. Gatchel, 276-298. New York: Guilford Press.

Romano, J., and J. A. Turner. 1985. Chronic pain and depression: Does the evidence support a relationship? *Psychological Bulletin* 97(1):18-34.

Rome, J. D., C. O. Townsend, B. K. Bruce, C. D. Sletten, C. A. Luedtke, and J. E. Hodgson. 2004. Chronic noncancer pain rehabilitation with opioid withdrawal: Comparison of treatment outcomes based on opioid use status at admission. *Mayo Clinical Proceedings* 79(6):759-768.

Rosensteil, A., and F. J. Keefe. 1983. The use of coping strategies in chronic low back pain patients: Relationship to patient characteristics and adjustment. *Pain* 17(1):33-43.

Schmidt, A. J. M. 1985a. Cognitive factors in the performance of chronic low back pain patients. *Journal of Psychosomatic Research* 29(2):183-189.

———. 1985b. Performance level of chronic low back pain patients in different treadmill test conditions. *Journal of Psychosomatic Research* 29(6):639-646.

Schoefferman, J. 1994. The use of medications for pain of spinal origin. Paper presented at "The Final Link to Therapeutic Success" course, San Francisco.

Shealy, S., J. T. Mortimer, and J. B. Rewick. 1967. Electrical inhibition of pain by stimulation of the dorsal columns. *Anesthesia and Analgesia* 46(4):489-491.

Spiegel, D., and J. R. Bloom. 1983. Pain in metastatic breast cancer. *Cancer* 52(2):341-345.

Sternbach, R. A. 1983. *How Can I Learn to Live with Pain When It Hurts So Much?* Unpublished.

Sullivan, M. J. L., B. Thorn, J. A. Haythornthwaite, F. Keefe, M. Martin, L. A. Bradley, and J. C. Lefebvre. 2001. Theoretical perspectives on the relation between catastrophizing and pain. *Clinical Journal of Pain* 17(1):52-64.

Tearnan, B. H., and M. J. Lewandowski. 1992. The Behavioral Assessment of Pain Questionnaire: The development and validation of a comprehensive self-report instrument. *American Journal of Pain Management* 2(4):181-191.

Travell, J. G., and D. G. Simons. 1992. *Myofascial Pain and Dysfunction: The Trigger Point Manual.* Baltimore: Williams and Wilkins.

Turk, D. C., and E. S. Monarch. 2002. Biopsychosocial perspective on chronic pain. In *Psychological Approaches to Pain Management: A Practitioner's Handbook*, ed. D. C. Turk and R. J. Gatchel, 3-29. New York: Guilford Press.

Turk, D. C., and F. Winter. 2006. *The Pain Survival Guide: How to Reclaim Your Life*. Washington, DC: American Psychological Association.

Von Korff, M., and K. Saunders. 1996. The course of back pain in primary care. *Spine* 21(24):2833-2837.

Waddell, G., M. Newton, I. Henderson, D. Sommerville, and C. J. Main. 1993. A Fear-Avoidance Beliefs Questionnaire (FABQ) and the role of fear-avoidance beliefs in chronic low back pain and disability. *Pain* 52(2):157-168.

Waddell, G., and D. C. Turk. 1992. Clinical assessment of low back pain. In *Handbook of Pain Assessment*, ed. D. C. Turk and R. Melzack, 15-36. New York: Guilford Press.

Wesley, A. L., R. J. Gatchel, J. P. Garofalo, and P. B. Polatin. 1999. Toward more accurate use of the Beck Depression Inventory with chronic back pain patients. *Clinical Journal of Pain* 15(2):117-121.

Williams, D. A., and F. J. Keefe. 1991. Pain beliefs and the use of cognitive-behavioral coping strategies. *Pain* 46(2): 185-190.

Blake H. Tearnan, Ph.D., is director of behavioral medicine for the Functional Restoration Program at Washoe Medical Center Rehabilitation Hospital in Reno, and clinical director for the Southern Nevada Functional Restoration Program in Las Vegas, NV. He graduated from the University of Georgia's Clinical Psychology Program with a specialization in clinical and medical psychology. He has held positions at the University of Wisconsin, University of Nevada Medical School, and the Veterans Affairs Medical Center in Reno, NV. He was also clinical coordinator at the Sierra Pain Institute and director of the Sonora Pain Center. Tearnan is a founding partner of the Reno Spine Center, president of HealthNetSolutions.com, and a consultant to various groups including Innovative Health Solutions and the American Academy of Pain Management, where he is on the board of advisors.

Tearnan has published widely in the areas of medical rehabilitation, health, pain, and anxiety disorders. He is the author of numerous psychometric instruments on general health, pain, and disability including the Pain Disability Report, Behavioral Assessment of Pain, and the Life Assessment Questionnaire.

more **real tools** for coping with chronic pain
from new**harbinger**publications

LIVING BEYOND YOUR PAIN
Using Acceptance & Commitment Therapy to
Ease Chronic Pain

$19.95 • Item Code: 4097

THE TRIGGER POINT THERAPY WORKBOOK,
SECOND EDITION
Your Self-Treatment Guide for Pain Relief

$19.95 • Item Code: 3759

THE FROZEN SHOULDER WORKBOOK
Trigger Point Therapy for Overcoming Pain &
Regaining Range of Motion

$18.95 • Item Code: 447X

FIBROMYALGIA & CHRONIC FATIGUE SYNDROME
7 Proven Steps to Less Pain & More Energy

$14.95 • Item Code: 4593

10 SIMPLE SOLUTIONS TO MIGRAINES
Recognize Triggers, Control Symptoms
& Reclaim Your Life
$12.95 • Item Code: 4410

available from new**harbinger**publications
and fine booksellers everywhere

To order, call toll free **1-800-748-6273** or visit our online bookstore at **www.newharbinger.com**
(V, MC, AMEX • prices subject to change without notice)